THE RISKS OF PRESCRIPTION DRUGS

D1249203

The Columbia University Press and Social Science Research Council
Series on the Privatization of Risk

THE COLUMBIA UNIVERSITY PRESS AND
SOCIAL SCIENCE RESEARCH COUNCIL
SERIES ON THE PRIVATIZATION OF RISK

Edited by Craig Calhoun and Jacob S. Hacker

The early twenty-first century is witnessing a concerted effort to privatize risk—to shift responsibility for the management or mitigation of key risks onto private-sector organizations or directly onto individuals. This series uses social science research to analyze this issue in depth. Each volume presents a concise review of a particular topic from the perspective of the public and private allocation of risk and responsibility and offers analysis and empirical, evidence-based opinion from leading scholars in the fields of economics, political science, sociology, anthropology, and law. Support for the series comes from the John D. and Catherine T. MacArthur Foundation.

Jacob S. Hacker, ed., *Health at Risk: America's Ailing Health System—and How to Heal It*

Andrew Lakoff, ed., *Disaster and the Politics of Intervention*

Katherine S. Newman, ed., *Laid Off, Laid Low: Political and Economic Consequences of Employment Insecurity*

Mitchell A. Orenstein, ed., *Pensions, Social Security, and the Privatization of Risk*

Robert E. Wright, ed., *Bailouts: Public Money, Private Profit*

The Risks of
Prescription Drugs

EDITED BY DONALD W. LIGHT

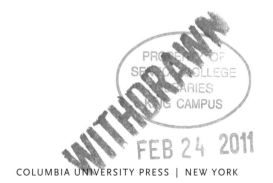

COLUMBIA UNIVERSITY PRESS | NEW YORK

A COLUMBIA/SSRC BOOK

COLUMBIA UNIVERSITY PRESS
Publishers Since 1893
New York   Chichester, West Sussex

Copyright © 2010 The Social Science Research Council

Library of Congress Cataloging-in-Publication Data

The risks of prescription drugs / edited by
Donald W. Light.
    p. cm.—(The Columbia University Press
and Social Science Research Council series on the
privatization of risk) (Columbia/SSRC book)
   Includes bibliographical references and index.
   ISBN 978-0-231-14692-0 (cloth : alk. paper)—
ISBN 978-0-231-14693-7 (pbk. : alk. paper)—
ISBN 978-0-231-51926-7 (ebook)
   1. Pharmaceutical policy—United States.
2. Pharmaceutical industry—Risk management.
3. Drugs—Risk factors. 4. United States. Food and Drug
Administration. I. Light, Donald, 1942– II. Series:
Columbia University Press and Social Science Research
Council series on the privatization of risk. III. Series:
Columbia/SSRC book.
   [DNLM: 1. Drug Industry—standards—United
States. 2. Prescription Drugs—standards—United
States. 3. Drug Toxicity—United States. 4. Medication
Errors—prevention & control—United States. 5. Risk
Assessment—United States. QV 736 R5955 2010]

RA401.A3R57 2010
338.4'76151—dc22

2010009014

Design by Julie Fry
Cover by Vin Dang

CONTENTS

Something is very wrong with a system that leads patients to demand, and doctors to prescribe, a drug that provides no better relief and causes significantly more serious side effects... How have we gotten to a place where expensive new drugs could become "blockbusters" when there was little scientific evidence to justify their routine use?
— John Abramson, MD, 2004

THE RISKS OF PRESCRIPTION DRUGS

CHAPTER ONE

Bearing the Risks of Prescription Drugs

DONALD W. LIGHT

Americans live in an era of advanced medicine in which many of the risks from pathogens and disease are controlled by prescription drugs. Each year, one or two excellent new drugs enable more people to lead healthier lives. These have built up to an impressive medicine chest of beneficial drugs. Despite this record of success, the fact remains that most new drugs pharmaceutical companies develop offer few advantages over existing ones and yet bear greater risk.

The benchmark for the U.S. Food and Drug Administration (FDA) to approve a drug as effective is evidence that it is better than, or no worse than, a placebo or inactive substance.[1] New drugs are compared only "occasionally with an existing drug for the condition."[2] As we will see in the next section, studies over the past 40 years have found that most new drugs offer few clinical advantages over existing ones. Thus, when ads or articles claim that a new drug is "more effective" or "better," the question to ask is, "Compared to what?"

When the FDA approves new drugs as "safe," the agency depends on company-run clinical trials. Pharmaceutical companies have an interest in designing trials to maximize evidence of effectiveness over placebos and to minimize evidence of adverse reactions. The more recent speed-up in FDA review times negotiated by the pharmaceutical industry in return for subsidizing the FDA's drug approval process has resulted in the prescription of many newer drugs that subsequently prove dangerous enough to end up requiring warnings, restrictions, or removal from the market.[3]

Patients are exposed to greater risk for hidden side effects as the public body designed to protect them approves new drugs as "safe and effective" that, from a clinical or patient's point of view, may not be either. Chapter 2 will describe the long struggle to protect consumers from toxic drugs and recent efforts by Congress to reform the FDA to enhance public protection. How well this reform will reduce patient risk is unclear because the FDA is so intimately tied to the industry it is supposed to regulate.

Because most new drugs offer little or no advantage over existing drugs to offset their greater risk, patients who take them may put themselves at greater risk than if they took an older, safer drug at much less cost. The incidence of serious adverse effects is significant. A review of studies in 1998 concluded that "overall 2,216,000 hospital patients experienced a serious ADR (adverse drug reaction) in the United States in 1994."[4] An estimated 106,000 died, making adverse drug reactions the fourth leading cause of death, behind stroke but ahead of pulmonary disease and accidents.[5] The authors called the rates "extremely high." Applying the same rates to the most recent census data projects 2,335,000 ADRs among hospitalized patients and 111,136 deaths in 2006.[6] Risks increase with age as the ability of the kidney and liver to excrete drugs declines. Starfield, in a wider review of adverse effects, concludes that at least 225,000 patients die each year from all forms of medicine in a system prone to fragmented, excessive treatment.[7]

Adverse drug reactions reported to the FDA nearly tripled between 1995 and 2005, from 156,000 to 460,000 (figure 1.1).[8] A decade earlier, in 1985, only 38,000 reports were submitted. According to Public Citizen, 1.5 million Americans a year are hospitalized due to adverse drug reactions.[9] If Americans consume about 40% of all drugs in the world, this would mean 3.75 million hospitalizations worldwide. Between 1998 and 2005, reported serious adverse events increased four times faster than the total number of outpatient prescriptions. These studies each have their limitations, but together they indicate how substantial are the risks that patients bear.

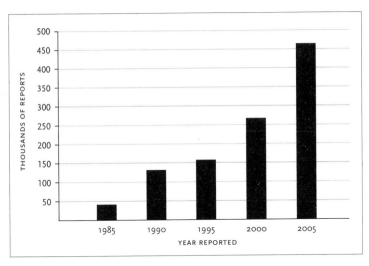

Figure 1.1 Adverse drug event reports to FDA [Source: Adapted from FDA, CDER "Report to the Nation: Improving Public Health through Human Drugs," 2005, p. 37]

There is no sign of the increase leveling out. Assuming a constant reporting rate, ADRs are rising about 15% each year, and a shift to biologics as safer because more "natural" is offering no relief. A study of the new biologics has found that safety-related regulatory action was taken on 14% of them within the first three years on the market and 29% within the first 10 years.[10] Seventy percent of the serious side effects were identified within the first five years of use, and the other 30% in the next five years. First-in-class (breakthrough) biologics were 3.7 times more likely to result in a safety warning than biologics in existing classes.[11]

There are good reasons to believe that toxic side effects are even more widespread than the figures above. Former FDA Commissioner David Kessler has written that "only about 1% of serious events are reported to the FDA," and the FDA Office of Drug Safety believes only 1% of ADRs are reported,[12] which for 2005 would mean about 46 million adverse drug reactions.

The review of studies did not count ADRs due to overdose, errors in drug administration, and other factors that are extrinsic to the drugs themselves; rather the review found an emphasis on high dosages throughout the current system, massive commercial promotion, and the use of brand names that look or sound similar.[13] These include a substantial number of young adults 18–25 who take psychotherapeutic drugs, stimulants, and sedatives obtained outside the regulated market for non-medical uses.[14] Many researchers also do not count serious ADRs or deaths in nursing homes or anywhere outside hospitals. More important are the factors that the prize-winning *New York Times* journalist Melody Petersen identifies in her book *Our Daily Meds*.[15] When drugs make patients dizzy, resulting in a bad fall, or drowsy, resulting in a car accident, or less able to fight off a serious illness because of a weakened immune system, official reports cite the bad fall, the car accident, or the new disease, not the underlying problem of drug side effects. Petersen reports that doctors who fill out death certificates are instructed to call a "therapeutic misadventure" a natural death. The role of a drug in a heart attack or stroke or in liver failure is usually not noted. Yet when pathologists have investigated liver failure cases more thoroughly, for example, they have found that 51% were caused by just one active ingredient, acetaminophen, which is sold as Tylenol and is combined with many other drugs.[16] Petersen cites other in-depth studies that find drugs as an underlying cause of death in which the prescribing doctor is often the one who fills out the death certificate.

The number of prescriptions increased 72% from 1997 to 2007, much faster than increased illness due to aging or other factors.[17] More people are taking drugs longer, for months or years, and the risk of side effects rises with length of use. In addition, the risk of drug interactions increases rapidly as a patient takes more drugs. There can be a *cascade effect*, as additional drugs are prescribed to deal with the harmful side effects of initially prescribed drugs, these may also generate their own side effects. For all these reasons, the individualized risk of taking prescription drugs is probably much larger than estimates based on hospitalized patients. Patients may reasonably expect the FDA and their physician to protect them from risk, but in fact, both pass significant risk on to patients.

This book describes how the privatization of medical risk has grown with the ever-increasing ingestion of drugs for more and more conditions, many with questionable clinical basis and approved by a regulatory system that often fails to provide adequate risk protection. Medical doctors and social scientists describe in these pages how the current system of developing, testing, approving, and dispensing drugs relies more on marketing than good science, especially through the market-based construction of new diseases or medical conditions, such as high cholesterol (Chapter 3), mental "illnesses" (Chapter 4), and menopause (Chapter 5). Adverse drug reactions are part of a larger pattern of avoidable injuries and deaths resulting from a fragmented health care system that concerned critics believe leads to overtreatment and non-beneficial prescriptions.[18] Overtreatment and rising prices also put millions at financial risk.[19]

TRADEOFFS BETWEEN BENEFITS AND HARMS

On average, most new drugs offer little or no additional benefit over existing drugs to offset their risks. A careful review of therapeutic benefits and harms for each new drug over the past two decades has concluded that 2–3% are real breakthroughs and another 11% offer some advantage over existing drugs, for a total of 14%, or one in seven.[20] In the 1960s and 1970s, when the FDA used to rate the therapeutic contributions of new drugs precisely, it judged 2.1% of 1,861 drug candidates as therapeutic breakthroughs and 8.6% as modestly superior.[21] Together these indicate that one in nine new drugs offer a modest or significant therapeutic gain, the same ratio that an often-cited industry assessment found for all internationally marketed drugs from 1975 to 1994.[22] Thus for over 40 years, most new drugs have offered few advantages to offset risks, and only a small proportion have provided real clinical advantages over existing ones.[23]

Those 11–14% of new drugs that offer real therapeutic advantages have helped millions of patients, and if there are two or three new ones a year, they add up over time to a significant arsenal against disease and death. Further, several of the 86–89% that are little or no better on average can help some patients who have a different biogenetic make-up. Most companies, however, focus on mass marketing and devote most of their R&D funds to filling or replacing their product line with newly patented drugs that can be priced higher but offer few advantages to offset the greater risks.[24] Pharmaceutical company reports show they spend only 1.3% of sales revenues for basic research to discover new drugs, net of taxpayers' subsidies.[25] Increasingly, the big companies do less research to discover new drugs and let thousands of research labs and biotechnology firms try to find promising new products, then buy in and focus on marketing them. They spend about three times more on marketing than on market-oriented "research," and only a small percentage of that research is basic.

The Health Research Group at Public Citizen has been primarily concerned about drug safety for 30 years and is funded by subscriptions and donations. It has identified more than 180 approved drugs that are too toxic for patients to take. In many cases the FDA approved them despite evidence of serious risks or little advantage over other drugs. They include such well-known products as Bextra, Celebrex, Crestor, Lamisil, Levitra, and Singulair, some of which had warnings added or were withdrawn after the Health Research Group advised against them.[26] The Group is constantly petitioning the FDA to ban further dangerous drugs, like the widely used drug for diabetes, Avandia.[27]

Many patients also receive unnecessary or inappropriate drugs. For example, in a detailed study of all the medications taken by elderly patients admitted to a university hospital in France, two-thirds had been given at least one inappropriate medication, and 20% of them had an ADR.[28] Almost as many (16.4%) taking *appropriate* medications had a toxic drug reaction too. Would the results be as pervasive in American university hospitals?

In weighing trade-offs, the interests of drug companies and patients differ sharply. Pharmaceuticals is a high-risk industry that routinely develops new products with toxic side effects — products that often fail. Executives therefore deal with risk all the time and have a long history of trying out potentially beneficial drugs to "see what happens."[29] They want quick approvals to get drugs out into the market. Companies budget for the costs of adverse effects and lawsuits for damages as routine. They pay millions to settle claims against toxic side effects and seal the evidence and millions more to settle claims for deceptive advertising, then keep on marketing.[30] Before testing for safety was required, some pharmaceutical companies put drugs on the market without testing them, as described in Chapter 2, though others were more cautious and responsible.

Patients, by contrast, have one body and want to avoid any risk to it. Thus there is an inherent clash of two cultures: a high-risk business trying to sell any drugs they can[31] and no-risk patients who want every drug to be safe, even if they know that is unrealistic. But patients also want to feel better, get treatment, and avoid future illness.

To say that new drugs are tested to be "safe" is misleading. When any drug is approved, the most one can say is that it is "apparently safe based on partial information."[32] The usual emphasis is on how rare side effects cannot be known from clinical trials that involve 1,000–3,000 subjects and often collect data over a short period of time. While true, "randomized trials" can be designed so more common adverse reactions are not reported by excluding many of the patients who will actually use a drug and ending a trial before many side effects arise. If trials were designed to test for safety, the risks to patients could be substantially reduced. In addition, risks of serious side effects are sometimes known while under review, and technical staff advise against exposing patients to them but are overruled.[33]

When pharmaceutical companies say a drug is "effective" or "more effective," they usually mean more effective than a placebo, not more effective than existing drugs. In fact, the FDA is not allowed to compare a new drug to drugs already on the market in considering approval. "More effective" also usually means more effective for treating a surrogate measure of the clinical risk or problem rather than the problem itself. For example, the rationale for statins, a class of drugs that lowers cholesterol, is based on the theory that lowering cholesterol (a soft, surrogate measure) reduces the risk of coronary heart disease (CHD, a hard, clinical measure). The theory is clearly supported for patients with a history of heart disease. But Howard Brody, a practicing physician and a distinguished professor of medical ethics, describes in Chapter 3 how commercially sponsored research, publications, professional conferences, professional education, and promotion have led physicians and otherwise healthy people with high cholesterol levels to believe that taking a statin will also reduce their risk of CHD. Yet the picture of benefits and harms for statins varies by gender, age, and pre-existing risks, and studies cited for guidelines to prescribe statins do not support them.[34] Millions of people taking statins may not be obtaining any benefit from the drug.

Even the widely accepted practice of lowering blood sugar in type 2 diabetics to prevent heart disease, stroke, and kidney failure is being questioned by newer evidence and some experts. In February 2008, NIH stopped a large trial testing drugs to lower blood sugar in type 2 diabetics because the death rate from all causes was *higher* among those taking medication than in the control group. A second large trial found no clinical benefits from diabetes drugs as well as some additional adverse outcomes, such as severe hypoglycemia.[35] Soft, surrogate end points are used in clinical trials on the assumption that lowering blood sugar has a clinical benefit that outweighs the risks in type 2 diabetes. A recent study at the Cleveland Clinic, however, challenges this assumption for one class of anti-diabetic drugs, which includes Actos®, Avandia® (rosiglitazone), and Rezulin® (troglitazone, which is no longer marketed due to liver toxicities). In fact, the Cleveland Clinic meta-analysis of many clinical trials suggests that these drugs actually increase patient risk of a cardiovascular event; yet millions of people are still taking them.[36]

THE INSTITUTIONALIZATION OF HOPE AND MAGIC

The rules and practices by which so many new drugs of little benefit and real risk get approved and marketed reflect the hope and optimism that characterize American culture.[37] Fears and uncertainties about symptoms and illnesses foster magical thinking. The doctor-patient relationship and medicine more generally center around institutionalized roles of improvement and hope, even though the majority of illness today is chronic and more illness comes with age. The physician is expected "to 'do everything possible' to achieve the complete, early and painless recovery of his patients," though often not much can be done.[38] Such magical expectations put physicians under strain because evidence of effectiveness is based on probabilities, the course of a given patient's illness is uncertain, and how an individual patient will react is also uncertain. Prescribing a drug becomes like a ritual of hope and magical healing in the face of fear and uncertainty. Beyond the statistic that six in every seven new drugs offer little or no clinical advantage over other treatments, many patients do not respond to the benefit of a given drug because of their biogenetic make-up, while others respond well.

Executives and marketers know their anthropology. They have developed some of the most elaborate institutions of hope and magic in modern culture, tended to by marketing experts, medical writers, leading clinicians on retainer, paid educators, and journalists. Doctors and patients do not want to hear that new magic potions are dangerous or no better. Sales reps tell physicians what they want to hear, that a new product bears hope, not harm. They leave free samples, which physicians can bear as gifts to their patients, along with the message that this new medicine has stronger magic than the older ones. Uncertainty, anxiety, and fear melt away. Parsons even wrote in 1951: "...pseudo-science is the functional equivalent of magic in the modern medical field."[39]

DO PHYSICIANS PROTECT PATIENTS FROM RISK?

When the FDA began to require a doctor's prescription for most new drugs in the 1940s, it passed on more of the responsibility for protecting patients from the regulator to physicians.[40] But physicians are often too busy to read through all the journals and do not use independent sources like *The Medical Letter* to assess the pros and cons of newer drugs. Instead, they get their information from friendly, generous sales reps who tend to emphasize the benefits and minimize the risks of prescribing their newest products for ever-expanding indications.[41] In addition, more than three-quarters of physicians have received favors from drug companies whose brands they prescribe, and almost one-third have developed personal relations with sales reps.[42] Highly priced drugs for cancer have led some companies to pay "rebates," or kickbacks, for prescribing more of their drug, amounting to nearly $800 million to oncologists in 2006 alone and leading to dangerous overprescribing.[43] The Senate Finance Committee and leading investigative journalists have found a still wider pattern of companies paying large sums to leading clinicians to promote diseases, broaden the criteria for their diagnosis, and promote patented drugs to treat them.[44] The upshot for patients when they agree to take a drug is uninformed consent, or even misinformed consent.

Most of the continuing education for practicing physicians is sponsored by pharmaceutical companies, often under generous terms and in five-star locations.[45] Through market-driven research that signs up prescribers as "investigators," publications, educational programs, and one-on-one promotion, companies give physicians every reason to prescribe more drugs to more patients, which inadvertently exposes them to still more toxic side effects.[46]

In a UCLA study with taped transcripts of office visits, two-thirds of the time physicians failed to mention harmful side effects of the drugs they were prescribing.[47] In another recent study, half the patients on statins who complained of muscle aches, pain, memory lapses, or cognitive impairments were told by their doctors that their problems were not related to their statins.[48] The doctors said the symptoms were in their patient's imagination, or they could not be due to statins, even though medical studies showed all these toxic side effects are found in patients taking statins. Although they probably do not see it this way, physicians provide the perfect cover for drug companies: rather than serving as a trusted protector of their patients, they prescribe without mentioning adverse reactions and then dismiss them when they arise.

THE FDA: PROTECTING INDIVIDUALS FROM RISK?

The FDA is charged with ensuring that benefits outweigh risks of harm, and the extensive though flawed testing system overseen by the agency does weed out a large number of drug candidates that would cause more harm than good if they were approved. Yet the FDA still approves some drugs that put patients at risk of toxic side effects, and this trend seems to have increased in recent years.[49] Pressure from pharmaceutical companies and underfunding by Congress, as explained more fully in Chapter 2, led to industry becoming the major funder of FDA reviews of new drugs in return for setting faster review times.[50] This has led to increased risks of hidden side effects for patients, with billions of dollars spent persuading physicians to prescribe new drugs.[51] More new drugs are approved first in the United States and more quickly than anywhere else in the world; thus Americans are more exposed than patients in other countries to the risks of new drugs, as well as to their new benefits.

Prescription drugs may appear to be safe—doubly safe—because they have been prescribed by a physician and approved by the FDA. But the FDA's ability to protect people from hidden risks of serious harm has been compromised since "The Great Risk Shift"[52] of deregulation and the growth of the influence of pharmaceutical companies. Drug companies complain that FDA standards for safety and efficacy have become too stringent and costly. They point out that they do their own extensive testing and can be trusted to market drugs that are safe and effective. But as we will see in Chapter 2, some companies have tested minimally for safety on their own, until testing requirements were developed. They submit test data and assessments of risks that reviewers consider inadequate, and they usually fail to carry out post-marketing studies on safety as required by agreements in the approval process.

Although only one in seven new drugs offers a therapeutic advantage, about two in seven appear to result in enough serious adverse events to prompt the FDA to require a label change, though the FDA does not track this basic statistic.[53] The chances are about one in five that new drugs will eventually have warnings added that are so serious they are highlighted in a black box.[54] Label changes, however, underestimate the risks passed on to patients because the same division of the FDA that approves new drugs is responsible for subsequently deciding whether they are harming patients enough to recommend changes in use, issue warnings, or press companies to withdraw them. Besides their reluctance to admit a drug is less safe than they thought, officials have been required to seek company agreement on warnings. Often, FDA officers have recommended a warning, but months of negotiation-delayed responses from reluctant companies have resulted in watered-down statements that do not protect patients from the documented toxic effects.[55]

Research into the details of how the FDA approves drugs has found that it approves them with partial evidence of harmful effects or sometimes before the results of an important trial are in, and sometimes despite known risks, because it is under great pressure by companies and patients to get new drugs on the market.[56] The FDA increases risk this way through quick approvals that require post-approval trials, most of which are not completed.[57] The FDA Office of Drug Safety has limited staff or funds to monitor safety once drugs are on the market and few powers to restrict or withdraw a dangerous drug. It repeatedly recommends that dangerous drugs be taken off the market but is overruled by the body that approved them. The officers in charge are known to be both skeptical of the evidence coming in and reluctant to admit they approved a drug that is harming patients.[58]

This sketch of the FDA focuses principally on how its testing and approval fails to protect patients from risk, but there are other sources of risk not well protected by the FDA. For example, the active chemical ingredients of most "American" drugs have for years been manufactured abroad, mainly in China and India, where few plants are inspected by the FDA.[59]

A prominent case that illustrates patients' vulnerability to unmanageable risk in the current drugs system is Vioxx, an anti-inflammatory painkiller that almost no one needed because there were cheaper, safer alternatives at the time. David Graham, the associate director of the FDA Office of Drug Safety in 2004, called Vioxx "the single greatest drug safety catastrophe in the history of this country or the history of the world."[60] He estimated that Vioxx caused 88,000 to 130,000 heart attacks or strokes, with a mortality rate of 30–40%. The worldwide toll would be more than double that. Vioxx was the landmark case that led Congressmen to investigate why the FDA was not protecting patients better from risks and how so many people could suffer heart attacks, stroke, and death from taking just another anti-inflammatory painkiller.

Vioxx was claimed to halve stomach bleeds in the small percentage of people who experienced that risk when taking some kinds of common painkillers. Appropriately used, it would have been a second- or maybe third-line drug for that small group of patients. But a Congressional review documented how Merck aggressively marketed Vioxx for an ever-widening array of uses as the drug of first choice.[61] The sales reps hid or misrepresented the life-threatening side effects; this has been shown to be a general pattern.[62] Many of the "scientific" articles in medical journals attesting to the benefits of Vioxx were written by company-paid ghost writers, and academic researchers agreed to front as the authors.[63] Only a few physicians, like John Abramson, realized how articles in even the most respected journals spun incomplete and inaccurate evidence to hide the risks of both Celebrex and Vioxx while exaggerating their benefits.[64] Eric Topol, then chairman of cardiovascular medicine at the Cleveland Clinic, testified that the risks of cardiovascular trauma were known to the company since 1999 but hidden through "scientific misconduct" and said that Merck had attempted to "trash" doctors critical of Vioxx.[65]

Several seeding trials — clinical studies conducted by pharmaceutical companies that are primarily designed to fulfill marketing objectives — were set up by Merck's marketing department, even though they were opposed by Merck's own director of research as "intellectually redundant" and "dangerous" because they compromised the large clinically meaningful trials already done.[66] Market-driven trials, however, enable a company to pay leading clinicians to be part of the team, sign them up as champions, and then pay them speaker's fees to persuade colleagues to prescribe the new drug.

For example, Merck gave thousands of sales reps hundreds of millions of dollars to spend on physicians; the reps also provided tens of millions of free samples that physicians handed out to patients, which got them started taking Vioxx.[67] Some of these patients then began to experience heart attacks or strokes. This side effect was publicly known at least since 2001, when the FDA advisory committee report (along with the two graphs in figure 1.2) was posted on the Web—three years before Merck finally withdrew Vioxx.[68] Hard to understand, these two graphs showed that compared to Aleve (naproxen), Vioxx (rofecoxib) caused about one heart attack or stroke for every gastrointestinal bleed it avoided,[69] hardly what patients or their physicians were led to believe. Public Citizen warned patients not to use it. The *New York Times* published a front-page article in 2001 on the risks, but Merck countered with ads and materials attesting to the safety of Vioxx.[70] Merck completed a trial that demonstrated Vioxx's cardiovascular risk but did not report it to the FDA.[71] More physicians were persuaded to prescribe more Vioxx to more patients.

For many clinical and congressional leaders, Vioxx exemplified the failure of public safety agencies and a great risk shift to patients. Given that its cardio-traumatic effects were known early, why did the FDA not take more aggressive action? In fact it tried. Early on, FDA scientists identified how serious the risks were and put their findings on the Web.[72] Then FDA staff sent Merck executives a detailed and harsh letter with pages of examples of misleading claims in Merck's marketing campaign that overstated benefits and understated the risks to patients. They demanded that these misrepresentations stop. Like most such FDA letters, it was professional, tough, honest, and designed to protect patients. But all the solid work behind these warning letters is neutralized when companies take months to respond or circumvent them by slightly altering their marketing strategies (Chapter 5 offers an example of this practice in the case of hormone replacement therapy for women). In the Vioxx case, Merck made some adjustments in its promotional materials and continued its mass marketing.[73] Millions more patients continued to take it until Merck withdrew it in September 2004.

The Vioxx crisis and a rash of withdrawals of other new drugs ultimately resulted in a searching review by the Institute of Medicine,

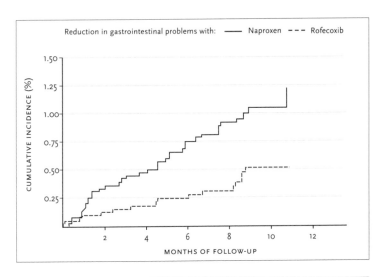

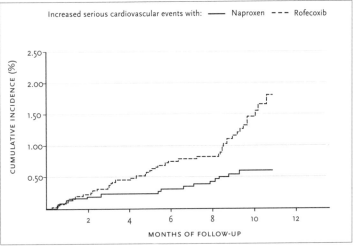

Figure 1.2   Evidence by February 2001 that Vioxx caused about one heart attack or stroke for every gastrointenstinal problem it prevented   [as originally presented by the FDA in February 2001]

numerous congressional hearings, and a detailed analysis of how the culture and organization of the FDA have marginalized staff who are concerned about safety and given them few powers to protect the public when clear signs of toxic side effects arise.[74] A number of new measures and changes are strengthening the FDA's ability to prevent another Vioxx, though fundamental weaknesses remain.

THE "RISK PROLIFERATION SYNDROME"

From my research, I have concluded that five institutional practices make up what could be called the risk proliferation syndrome: (1) having companies test their own products as part of a public regulatory system; (2) limiting reviewers' time so that they are unable to thoroughly assess the available data; (3) allowing mass marketing of new products when their safety is only partly known; (4) providing strong incentives to encourage unapproved uses; and (5) supporting the proliferation of new disease models that lack good evidence but lead millions of patients to take unnecessary drugs with their attendant risks.

CONFLICT-OF-INTEREST TESTING

The risk proliferation syndrome starts with a regulatory system that allows companies to test their own products and write up the results rather than requiring independent testing. Sponsoring companies have every reason to structure the tests, record what happens, analyze the data, and present results in ways that maximize evidence of benefits and minimize detection of risks. Minimum detection is achieved by a variety of techniques, such as:

- excluding patients who are older, poorer, minority, or female because they have more complex risk profiles and are more likely to suffer adverse effects;
- running short trials that record evidence of effectiveness but not toxic side effects that show up later, especially for higher dosages that are more effective but also bear more risk;
- running trials too small to pick up any but the most apparent, short-term toxic effects;
- recording only selected toxic side effects rather than all of them;
- ruling out patients with other health problems or risks, even if they are likely to be prescribed the drug once approved;
- using a comparator drug (if there is one) that has similar adverse effects so that the tested drug's risks do not stand out as statistically significant;

- excluding subjects who dropped out because they could not tolerate side effects, sometimes a large proportion;
- splitting clinically related adverse events into unique subgroups of one or two patients, such that none will be detected statistically;
- selectively publishing evidence to support marketing.

Other techniques include removing subjects who have a strong placebo response in a pre-trial dry run to reduce the placebo effect that the drug has to outperform; testing subjects before the trials begin and using only people who have a good response to the drug being tested; and secretly un-blinding the interim results midway through the trial "to see if they are sufficiently favorable" and then altering the design if needed before re-blinding the trial.[75]

Clinical trials have been increasingly contracted out to large for-profit companies that specialize in running trials that depend on good results to please their paymasters. An investigation found some contract research organizations advertise that they do scientifically valid research that will help prove the value of the products tested (a contradiction in terms), disguising their commercial nature in a number of ways.[76] A growing number of trials are conducted in developing countries where quality and ethical oversight are thin.[77] Based on the most detailed evidence we have, John Abraham concluded long ago that serious drug reactions are not an inevitable consequence of drug therapy but a consequence of how drug companies measure and interpret the data.[78]

Companies often design trials around patients with a principal condition who are otherwise healthy. For example, Merck ruled out patients with existing cardiovascular problems for critical trials of Vioxx, even though cardiovascular risks were "in the mechanism" of how the drug worked and may have been suspected from the beginning.[79] If the same companies that have invested millions to develop a drug also design the trials to test its safety and efficacy, we can expect them to use strategies like these to produce "scientific" evidence that they are safe and effective. The Office of the Inspector General repeatedly investigates conflict of interest (COI) and routinely finds that the FDA does not enforce regulations to protect the public from COI because there is an inherent conflict in having companies test their own products.

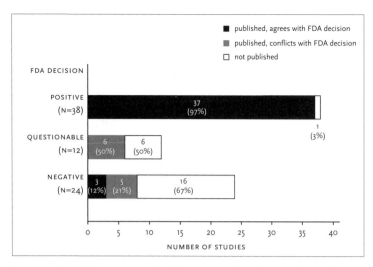

Figure 1.3   The misleading pattern of published evidence that a drug is safe and effective: 97% of antidepressant drug trials the FDA judged as positive were published in medical journals, compared to only 12% judged as negative [Source: Adapted from Erick H. Turner et al., "Selective Publication of Antidepressant Trials and Its Influence on Apparent Efficacy," *New England Journal of Medicine* 358 (2008): 252]

Sponsoring companies also engage in "ghost management" of research and publication to make it appear as if academic researchers are doing the studies and authoring scientific articles on the results.[80] Companies also manage what gets published and what does not. For example, one analysis found that 97% of antidepressant trials deemed positive by the FDA were published, whereas only 12% of trials with negative results were published and another 21% of the trials that the FDA judged to contain negative results were published so as to appear positive (see figure 1.3).[81] If the results from the negative trials are added to the published positive results, antidepressants are found to be barely more effective than placebos and to have serious side effects, a picture that was hidden for years.[82] Another review of generic and brand-name drugs for cardiovascular disease found that nearly all trials concluded they were equivalent, but half the editorials in medical journals counseled against using generics.[83]

A related bias in analysis and publication arises from not testing a hypothesis with trial data but doing scores of correlations and picking out the ones that are significant and favorable to the drug. Since one in every

20 will be "significant" at the 0.05 level by chance, one is sure to come up with "significant findings" that have no scientific validity. One expert calls this "the most insidious and misleading of the biases that affect this area of research...allowing the manipulation of data without any overt fraudulent action."[84] Senator Charles Grassley, as part of his investigations into drug company influence, wrote that "any attempt to manipulate the scientific literature, that can in turn mislead doctors to prescribe drugs that may not work and/or cause harm to their patients, is very troubling."[85] In response to the Vioxx crisis and subsequent investigations, Congress requires now that information about clinical trials and selected results be posted on ClinicalTrials.gov, "whatever their source of funding."[86] The World Health Organization and the International Committee of Medical Journal Editors also require that trial data be publicly registered. But registration is incomplete and delayed. Some results are required, but not toxic side effects, and no data on drugs that fail to be approved or are withdrawn. A loophole allows a two-year delay of posting trial data, and "the FDA must treat much of the data on clinical trials...as 'confidential commercial information.'" A senior reviewer concludes: "...the withholding of critical information about the safety and efficacy of marketed drugs from the public is unacceptable both ethically and scientifically."[87]

APPROVAL SPEED-UP

The pharmaceutical industry has used its well-funded lobbying organization to campaign for faster approvals to maximize sales and profits before patents run out. We have already cited evidence that this is increasing the risk of serious adverse side effects.[88] Companies continually complain that delays in approval and costly reviews slow down research. What patients need, the argument goes, is quicker approvals and faster access to new, better, and life-saving drugs. This may be true for a handful of medicines to treat patients for whom all available options have failed or where available treatments are themselves highly toxic. However, for the vast majority of new drugs, better data on risks and benefits, not rapid access, would mean lower risks for patients.

MASS MARKETING OF RISKY DRUGS

A third component of the risk proliferation syndrome consists of the regulations, practices, and institutions that encourage and carry out mass marketing after a drug has been approved rather than trying it out for a year on a limited and closely monitored population. "Greater access" is often code for mass marketing to get as many patients as possible on new drugs, which dilutes their benefits and spreads their risk of harm.

Marketing departments have been found repeatedly to understate or hide information about known risks, not only from patients but from their doctors. A Congressional review of marketing materials on Vioxx before it was withdrawn documents that each time a major report described its dangerous side effects, Merck redoubled its efforts to insist it was safe.[89] At this writing, Pfizer is pushing Chantix, its antismoking drug, during prime time news, even though side effects reported to the FDA exceeded reports for the ten best-selling drugs combined.[90] The total spent by companies on marketing is staggering—$57.5 billion,[91] far more than the small amount that companies spend on basic research to find better drugs.[92] One important technique is to promote expensive new drugs to hospital specialists and make them available at little or no cost so that patients start them before discharge. Another is to leave free samples of new drugs (total annual value of $16 billion) in doctors' offices to encourage initiation of treatment in outpatients. Once started, few patients feel comfortable switching to alternatives that are less risky and yet effective.

Direct-to-consumer advertising, or DTCA, plays a central role in "educating" millions of people to view their symptoms as signs of a medical problem, or future problem, that they need to treat. Expenditures for advertising products directly to the public rose from $985 million in 1995 to $4.2 billion in 2005, focused almost entirely on newly approved drugs with blockbuster potential (more than $1 billion in annual sales).[93] Yet many heavily advertised drugs offer no substantial advantages to patients over existing ones.[94] Real benefits can be small. For example, 30–50 people with high cholesterol but no other risk factors need to take a statin for five years in order for one heart attack to be avoided. If the chance of a heart attack is reduced from 3% to 2%, the drug can be promoted as cutting heart attacks by one-third rather than by 1%. Television ads only have to mention major risk information and can result in an unbalanced, favorable picture of risks to patients. Most FDA letters to companies regarding DTCA concern their minimizing risks or exaggerating effectiveness, or both. Viewers and patients are unlikely to know how they are being misled. At the same time, because they are tax-deductible, drug ads are subsidized by consumers; this has disturbed some members of Congress.[95]

In addition to direct-to-consumer advertising (DTCA), pharmaceutical marketing focuses on physician education during training, in the office, at conferences, and through continuing medical education courses.[96] These practices have led the Senate Finance Committee and the Senate Committee on Aging to hold hearings about industry influence on physician education and prescribing. Companies pay prominent specialists a few thousand dollars plus expenses to give educational seminars (often at expensive restaurants or luxurious resorts) about the best ways to treat a given clinical problem. In these ways a practicing physician is surrounded by facts, articles, courses, and sessions at specialty conferences that promote the use of new drugs as "more effective," even though 85% offer no advantage and may put patients at greater risk. In response, a number of reports, Congressional bills, and articles are strongly urging medical societies, medical centers, and physicians to sever ties with the industry in order to restore the trustworthiness of the profession.[97]

Pharmaceutical companies have colonized patient groups and health activists, providing them with "educational material," hand-picked speakers, and money.[98] Patient groups of serious diseases have become a principal lobbying force for faster approvals and insurance coverage for new drugs judged of marginal advantage by independent groups.

PROLIFERATING UNAPPROVED USES

Public regulation to protect patients from unsafe or ineffective drugs rests on the company selecting the indication for which a new drug is to be tested and then carefully designing and conducting trials to prove it is more effective than a placebo (or sometimes a comparator drug) for that indication. After approval, it is illegal for companies to market a drug for any condition or population in a manner inconsistent with the evidence of its specific effectiveness against specific conditions summarized in its label. However, this system is undermined by company-sponsored studies and trials in which clinicians are funded to try out a drug for other uses in small trials that often do not meet scientific standards.[99] These clinicians often publish the results in company-supported journals and supplements. They are also paid to give sponsored grand rounds, talks,

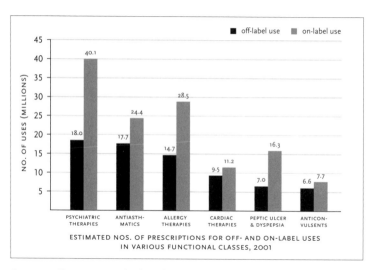

Figure 1.4 Physicians prescribe drugs for many unapproved uses [Source: Randall S. Stafford, "Regulating Off-Label Drug Use: Rethinking the Role of the FDA," *New England Journal of Medicine* 358 (2008): 1427]

educational courses, and conference presentations at which these publications are circulated as scientific-looking evidence for unapproved (off-label) uses or extensions of approved uses.

This system results in about one prescription in every five being written for an unapproved use, and in mental health, three out of every five antipsychotic drugs are prescribed for an unapproved use.[100] Yet three-fourths of the time the off-label uses have little or no scientific support.[101] Even when such off-label prescribing becomes substantial, companies are under no obligation to conduct scientifically rigorous studies to assess benefits and risks. Indeed, the short time left on the patent and possibility of identifying new risks are strong disincentives for not testing unapproved uses (figure 1.4). Why bother when one can get prominent physicians to promote them to their colleagues?

The FDA is not equipped to handle the large volume of marketing material that companies submit. Even when its small, underfunded staff identifies a serious risk, drafted letters have taken an average of seven months to be issued and longer to be enforced.[102] The Government Accounting Office found that the FDA received 277,000 submissions of marketing materials from 2003 to 2007, but its small staff could only get to 42 actions against off-label promotions. They could not say how many of the 277,000 promotional materials made off-label claims. A new rule allows sales reps to give physicians articles about off-label uses. Thus patients are not being protected by regulators from promotion for unapproved uses. This is a growing area of risks being put back on patients for uses that often have no proven off-setting benefit.

EXPANDING THE DOMAIN OF HEALTH PROBLEMS

Patient risks come not only from biased testing and the approval of drugs that have few advantages but also from companies and the experts they support promoting consumer acceptance of an ever-growing number of health problems or risks that drugs can fix.[103] Constructing new but dubious "diseases" creates new fears that call for hope and magic by opening new markets for products.[104] Mass screenings for real diseases or imagined risks produce large volumes of prescriptions or treatments that do not benefit patients.[105]

Ray Moynihan and Alan Cassels have researched several examples of commercially created or inflated illnesses resulting in overmedication.[106] One is high blood pressure. Blood pressure rises with age and is one of several factors that can increase the risk of heart attack or stroke. But because blood pressure is amenable to drugs, a world of marketing and guidelines developed around it. What constitutes "high" blood pressure is open to opinion, and U.S. guidelines set by expert panels have periodically lowered the criteria so that millions more people are labeled as "having hypertension," or now "prehypertension," and being "at risk" of heart disease. Nine of the eleven hypertension experts on the government panel that created the disease "prehypertension" had ties to the pharmaceutical industry, and nine of the twelve FDA panelists setting guidelines for blood pressure drugs had ties.[107] This corporate construction of personal risk feeds what has become a $40 billion market in blood pressure drugs.

Many other "diseases" could be added to the list of medical conditions treatable by prescription drugs. For example, the "epidemic" in obesity follows the classic sociological pattern of how a new problem is constructed by moral entrepreneurs, the press, and other interested parties.[108] Like high blood pressure and cholesterol, the definition of "obese" is lower than evidence of clinical danger. Another disorder afflicting millions is insomnia, based on the mythic eight-hour "good night's sleep" that has never been common. In 2007, the FDA issued a black box warning on the risks of taking all insomnia medicines. A review of evidence of benefits showed only seven out of every 100 patients on sleeping medications reported sleeping longer, by 25 minutes a night. Patient information leaflets mention only a fraction of all the risks to patients.[109] A third medical "disorder" that commercial interests are working hard to establish is "female sexual dysfunction," based on women reporting less than complete sexual fulfillment.[110]

The commercial construction of high cholesterol as a serious risk for heart disease has involved converting a complex set of relationships between heart disease and saturated fats and cholesterol in the diet and blood into a simple message that high cholesterol kills. Critics have been skeptical since the 1970s.[111] Recently, two major trials of statins found little evidence of reduced risk of heart attacks but increased total risk of morbidity and mortality, despite lower cholesterol.[112] Yet conflicting studies come out all the time; so the benefits of statins remain controversial. In 2008, the American Academy of Pediatrics recommended "more aggressive use of cholesterol-lowering drugs starting as early as the age of eight in hopes of preventing adult heart problems," despite growing evidence that lowering cholesterol has few clinical benefits.[113] The "high cholesterol kills" campaign and the research behind it are a good example of how approving any new drug better than an inert substance or placebo encourages the development of synthetic disease models based on surrogate measures. Another example is lowering blood sugar in type 2 diabetes to reduce heart disease.[114]

In Chapter 4, Allan Horwitz draws on his award-winning research into the basis for many of the official psychiatric diagnoses for non-psychotic patients[115] to describe the spectacular but dubious rise of attention deficit disorder, depression, and bipolar "disease." Increases in mental illness diagnoses have led to millions more people taking drugs whose main benefits are questionable, and serious side effects include addictive withdrawal symptoms and suicidal behavior, not to mention a neglect of the social causes of these emotional problems. Similarly, in Chapter 5, Cheryl Stults and Peter Conrad examine the development and impact of public "risk scares," as illustrated by turning menopause into a risk-laden medical condition that could cause Alzheimer's, osteoporosis, cardiovascular disease, and cancer. Hormone replacement therapy

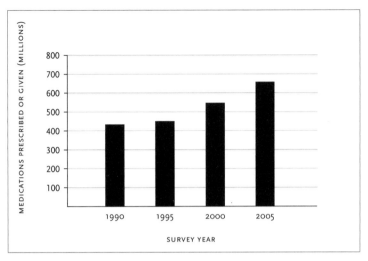

Figure 1.5   Medications prescribed or given during physician visits
[Source: National Ambulatory Medical Care Survey, United States, 1990–2005]

(HRT) was promoted for unproven benefits, and millions of women took it even though it did not reduce cardiovascular disease but significantly increased risk of breast cancer.[116] HRT is still promoted for these unproven benefits. Evidence from some of the 8,400 lawsuits by women who claimed to be damaged by Wyeth's hormonal drugs reveals details of how the company engaged ghost writers to publish twenty-six scientific papers supporting HRT and downplaying its side effects.[117]

As a result of convincing people they have more health problems and then urging them to take medication, approximately four-fifths of all Americans, including over half of all children, now take a prescription drug each week.[118] From 2000 to 2006, the number of people who reported taking five or more prescription medications doubled, and almost one in five adults over 65 years old take ten or more medications weekly.[119] The number of medications prescribed or given while seeing a physician rose from 425 to 679 million between 1990 and 2005, as shown in figure 1.5. The number of prescriptions rose 72% between 1997 and 2007.[120] The proliferation of "diseases" has contributed substantially to this increase.

Another contribution to risk proliferation is polypharmacy, the taking of multiple drugs for one or more conditions.[121] The toxic side effects of one drug lead doctors to prescribe another, which has its own risks and interactions that vary with the biological and genetic make-up of the individual. Since drugs are typically tested and approved as single entities, patients are put at risk for interactions. The proliferation of millions more people taking a second, third, or fourth drug multiplies the risk of serious adverse effects.

PATIENTS PUT AT FINANCIAL RISK

The risk proliferation syndrome puts more patients not only at greater clinical risk but also at greater financial risk. This volume is part of a project supported by the MacArthur Foundation and directed by the Social Science Research Council entitled "The Privatization of Risk." It concerns what Jacob Hacker called The Great Risk Shift that has taken place since 1980, away from job security, solid pensions, and health security toward putting individuals more at risk for their jobs, pensions, and health insurance.[122] This volume and the others address new questions about the ability of individuals to perceive, plan for, and successfully address these risks. Chapter 2 describes how regulations were developed to protect the public from serious risks from pharmaceuticals, how they were compromised, and the current efforts to protect the public from dangerous drugs like Vioxx.

The risk proliferation syndrome details a multi-pronged corporate effort to persuade physicians and their patients to buy new drugs that cost several times more than already existing drugs and often offer few clinical advantages to offset their risks of adverse reactions.[123] Private health insurance, for reasons explained in the companion volume, *Health at Risk*, puts many patients at greater financial risk than allowed by any country with universal health insurance.[124] For example, one in six Americans under age 65 *with* health insurance reports problems paying for a prescription. Among those without health insurance, nearly one in three report such problems. Most commercial policies cover drugs, but with deductibles, co-payments, caps, and gaps in drugs covered. These techniques for putting patients at greater financial risk are used much less in other countries. They force millions of Americans to think twice about whether to fill a prescription their doctors think they need and to split pills, share prescriptions, or stop taking a drug—each of which creates new safety risks. Patented drugs in the U.S. cost about twice as much as in Europe. Companies are free to charge substantially higher prices than in other wealthy countries for patented drugs in "free" markets where there is little price competition among patented drugs.[125] Yet physicians do not usually discuss affordability and cost with patients.[126]

The financial situation has worsened with the recession, and Americans are cutting back on the number of prescription drugs they take because they cost too much out of pocket.[127] In patient focus groups, patients decide which prescriptions they can do without. These choices take place in a context of Americans taking 72% more prescriptions in 2007 than a decade earlier, not because they are sicker but because of the risk proliferation syndrome that promotes fear of getting sick or worse and hope in new drugs.[128] Millions have benefited greatly from the medicine chest of good drugs that have been discovered one by one over the years; but millions more are put at financial and clinical risk by the proliferation of new drugs that offer few advantages but greater risks than older ones. Employers and insurers have responded by encouraging generic substitution through tiered co-payments.

MEDICARE'S DRUG COVERAGE RAVINE

Medicare was passed in 1964 after years of effort to reduce the great financial burden that seniors faced because insurance policies were either not available or unaffordable. The legislation did not cover the cost of most drugs, which has been increasing rapidly, from about $8 billion in 1970 to $40 billion in 1990 to $217 billion in 2006.[129] Although seniors were put at increasing financial risk, the pharmaceutical industry lobbied hard against proposals for Medicare to cover drug costs until seniors organized such a groundswell of protest over the high prices of drugs that it became a leading issue for both parties in the 2000 Congressional elections.[130] When work began on expanding Medicare coverage to drugs, the pharmaceutical industry and insurance companies made sure the terms included new multibillion dollar payouts for insurers and no discounts on patent-protected prices for drug companies.[131] Working under budget limitations, Congress decided that the only Medicare prescription program that would be acceptable must have some initial coverage for everyone and catastrophic coverage for people with very high drug expenses, leaving a ravine of no coverage in between.

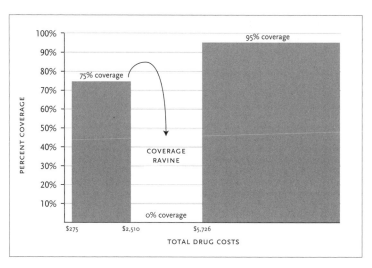

Figure 1.6   Medicare drug coverage ravine 2008 [Source: author]

The front edge of the coverage ravine in 2008 was $2,510 in drug costs (see figure 1.6), about the equivalent of one year's prescription for a patented drug costing $210 a month. Out-of-pocket costs add up to nearly half that total—a $275 deductible and 25% reimbursement for the remaining $2235 plus $610 on average for the premium. As shown in figure 1.6, patients stay in the ravine of no coverage until their bills exceed $5,726 out of pocket, plus monthly premiums for the policy that is giving them no reimbursement. At that point, they are hoisted up to the back safe ledge of 95% coverage. Thus a patient with a second medication costing $210 a month will pay all of it out of pocket so that both drugs cost her $5020 cash, unthinkable in other advanced industrial countries.

About one in five Medicare enrollees fall into the ravine of no coverage, and it will widen over time. It leaves millions of seniors paying thousands of dollars a year for costly drugs that are often little better than much cheaper ones because the drug lobby persuaded Congress to prohibit Medicare from negotiating volume discounts and because of overhead costs for the confusing extra layer of over 1,000 different drug benefit plans.[132] Consumers Union and AARP are especially concerned about large price increases of specialty drugs.[133] If Medicare could pay Canadian prices (an average of European prices) or negotiate for the same prices paid by the Veterans Health Administration, the heavy burden of zero coverage in the ravine between $2,510 and $5,726 could be filled in with coverage.[134] If Medicare paid Medicaid prices, much of the ravine could be filled. The industry claims that lower prices would reduce their funding for research to discover new, innovative drugs, but their own reports show they recover all research and other costs, plus a good profit from domestic sales in England and Canada.[135] Moreover, public funds pay for 84.2% of basic research to discover new drugs, and federal law has required since 1980 that products resulting from federally funded research must be "available to the public on reasonable terms." This law has not been enforced.[136]

Medicare also makes drug coverage an option, not automatic as in most countries. By requiring private plans, it incurs substantial costs for running them, which enrollees pay through drug plan premiums — another way in which the cost of drugs is increased for individuals. Four million eligible seniors do not enroll to avoid the costs and complexities. Overall, Medicare and Medicaid (which covers only half the poor, who also are sicker) leave millions to bear a significant financial burden when they become ill. Drug revenues are projected to rise from $217 billion in 2006 to $515 billion by 2017.

The personal financial burden of prescription drugs comes not only from taking more drugs than necessary but also from taking high-priced patented drugs that are usually little or no better than lower-priced generics, because the pharmaceutical industry spends billions on physicians to persuade them to prescribe the high-priced options. This personal burden is increased by toxic side effects and the costs for treating them — trips to the doctor or ER, more drugs to counter the side effects of the first drug, or hospitalization. On the other hand, the underinsured and uninsured may jeopardize their health by not taking drugs they need or stretching them out in ways that undermine their effectiveness.

The epilogue discusses ways to reduce the clinical and financial risks that patients now bear, beginning with no longer rewarding companies for developing new drugs of little therapeutic benefit but instead rewarding them for clinically superior new drugs. If this were done, then all new drugs would be worth considering, deceptive marketing that attempts to convey equivalent drugs as "better" would end, and there would be real clinical benefits to offset risks. The whole science of pharmaceutical research would improve because creating artificial diseases and disease models would no longer be rewarded. Employers, state governments, and insurers would save billions by not purchasing expensive new drugs that are not therapeutically superior. And if Congress funded the NIH to run or oversee clinical trials, we would not only get better information at an earlier stage about risks but industry would be relieved of a huge financial burden, eliminating the justification of pricing drugs at 50–100 times costs. Pharmaceuticals would no longer have to be a boom-and-bust business. The industry would become more stable, smaller, and rewarded for finding products that really improve people's health. These are just a few of several recommendations in the epilogue for Congress and the new administration to consider.

NOTES

1   FDA, *From Test Tube to Patient: The FDA's Drug Review Process: Ensuring Drugs Are Safe and Effective*, 4th edition, 2006, http://www.fda.gov/fdac/special/testtubetopatient/drugreview.html.

2   Institute of Medicine, Committee on the Assessment of the US Drug Safety System, *The Future of Drug Safety: Promoting and Protecting the Health of the Public* (Washington, DC: National Academies Press, 2007), 34.

3   M. K. Olson, "Are Novel Drugs More Risky for Patients Than Less Novel Drugs?" *Journal of Health Economics* 23 (2004): 1135–58; D. Carpenter, E. J. Zucker, and J. Avorn, "Drug-Review Deadlines and Safety Problems," *New England Journal of Medicine* 358 (2008): 1354–61; 359: 96–98.

4   J. Lazarou et al., "Incidence of Adverse Drug Reactions in Hospitalized Patients," *Journal of American Medical Association* 279 (1998): 1200–05, 1202. Like all estimates of cause of death, these estimates are only best approximations, and the methodological literature is full of details about how causes of death or hospitalization are subject to misjudgment, inaccurate recording, misattribution, and bias — in this case against identifying drugs as contributing to serious outcomes.

5   See FDA, *Preventable Adverse Drug Reactions*, 2002, http://www.fda.gov/CDER/DRUG/drugReactions/default.htm. See Public Citizen, "Adverse Drug Reactions: How Serious Is the Problem and How Often and Why Does It Occur?" *Worst Pills, Best Pills Newsletter*, 2009, http://www.worstpills.org/public/page.cfm?op_id=4&print=1.

6   6.7% of 34,854,000 hospital discharges = 2,335,000 ADRs. 4.6% of 2,416,000 deaths

in 2006 = 111,136. http://www.census.gov/compendia/statab/tables/09s0169.pdf; http://www.census.gov/prod/2007pubs/08abstract/vitstat.pdf. Because deaths from pulmonary disease and accidents have increased more, adverse reactions from taking drugs that are supposed to make you healthier now rank sixth as a cause of death. Compare Lazarou's list of leading causes on page 1204 with the latest from Information Please (2004) at http://www.infoplease.com/ipa/A0005110.html. Lazarou et al. make clear that with 106,000 deaths, ADRs are the fourth leading cause of death and that if the lower 95% CI of 76,000 deaths is used, they would rank sixth.

7   B. Starfield, "Is US Health Really the Best in the World?" *Journal of the American Medical Association* 284 (2000): 483–85.

8   FDA, CEDR, "Report to the Nation: Improving Public Health Through Human Drugs (2005)," http://www.fda.gov/cder/reports/rtn/2005/rtn2005.PDF; T. Moore, M. Cohen, and C. Furberg, "Serious Adverse Drug Events Reported to the Food and Drug Administration, 1998–2005," *Archives of Internal Medicine* 167 (2007): 1752–59.

9   Public Citizen, "Adverse Drug Reactions."

10 T. J. Giezen et al., "Safety-Related Regulatory Actions for Biologicals Approved in the United States and the European Union," *Journal of American Medical Association* 300 (2008): 1887–96.

11 The ratio of possible harms to benefits should be called the harm-benefit ratio, not the risk-benefit ratio.

12 D. A. Kessler, "Introducing MedWatch," *Journal of the American Medical Association* 269 (1993): 2765–67; L. Marsa, "Is Your Medicine Making You Sick?" *Ladies Home Journal* 2008 (July): 88–101.

13 A valuable organization concerned about the adverse side effects of an aggressive, brand-name industry is the Institute for Safe Medication Practices, www.ismp.org.

14 See Substance Abuse and Mental Health Services Administration, U.S. Department of Health and Human Services, "SAMHSA's Latest National Survey on Drug Use and Health," http://www.oas.samhsa.gov/NSDUHlatest.htm.

15 Melody Petersen, *Our Daily Meds: How the Pharmaceutical Companies Transformed Themselves into Slick Marketing Machines and Hooked the Nation on Prescription Drugs* (New York: Farrar, Straus and Giroux, 2008), chap. 9.

16 The study was done by the U.S. Acute Liver Failure Study. See Petersen, *Our Daily Meds*, 296.

17 Kaiser Family Foundation, *Prescription Drug Trends*, Sept. 2008, http://www.kff.org/rxdrugs/upload/3057_07.pdf.

18 John Abramson, *Overdosed America: The Broken Promise of American Medicine* (New York: Harper-Collins, 2004); Shannon Brownlee, *Overtreated: Why Too Much*

Medicine Is Making Us Sicker and Poorer (New York: Bloomsbury, 2007); Howard
Brody, *Hooked: Ethics, the Medical Profession, and the Pharmaceutical Industry* (Lanham, MD: Rowman & Littlefield, 2007); HealthGrades, "Fourth Annual Patient
Safety in American Hospitals Survey (2008)," http://www.healthgrades.com/
media/DMS/pdf/PatientSafetyInAmericanHospitalsStudy2007.pdf.

19 L. E. Felland and J. D. Reschovsky, "More Nonelderly Americans Face Problems
Affording Prescription Drugs," Center for Studying Health System Change, 2009,
http://www.hschange.com/CONTENT/1039/.

20 Prescrire International, "A Look Back at Pharmaceuticals in 2006: Aggressive
Advertising Cannot Hide the Absence of Therapeutic Advances," *Prescrire International* 16 (2007): 80–86.

21 John Abraham, *Science, Politics and the Pharmaceutical Industry: Controversy and
Bias in Drug Regulation* (London: Routledge, 1995), 243.

22 P. E. Barral, *20 Years of Pharmaceutical Research Results Throughout the World: 1975–94*
(Paris: Rhone-Poulenc Rorer Foundation, 1996).

23 Since it was forced to drop its earlier rating system in the 1980s and use broader
criteria, the FDA has given a "priority" rating to far more drugs.

24 Marcia Angell, *The Truth about the Drug Companies* (New York: Random House,
2004); Merrill Goozner, *The $800 Million Pill: The Truth behind the Cost of New
Drugs* (Berkeley: University of California Press, 2004).

25 D. W. Light and J. Lexchin, "Foreign Free Riders and the High Price of US Medicines," *British Medical Journal* 331 (2005): 958–60, http://bioethics.upenn.edu/
people/?last=Light&first=Donald.

26 Public Citizen, *Worst Pills, Best Pills Newsletter*, S. Wolfe, ed., Washington, DC,
http://www.worstpills.org/.

27 Public Citizen Health Research Group, http://www.citizen.org/publications/
release.cfm?ID=7614.

28 M-L. Laroche et al., "Is Inappropriate Medication Use a Major Cause of Adverse
Drug Reactions in the Elderly?" *British Journal of Clinical Pharmacology* 63 (2007):
177–86.

29 See Chapter 2 and Petersen, *Our Daily Meds*.

30 Ibid.

31 John Braithwaite, *Corporate Crime in the Pharmaceutical Industry* (London: Routledge & Kegan Paul, 1984); Milton Silverman, *The Drugging of the Americas: How
Multinational Drug Companies Say One Thing About Their Products to Physicians
in the United States and Another Thing to Physicians in Latin America* (Berkeley:
University of California Press, 1976); M. Silverman, P. R. Lee, and M. Lydecker,

Prescriptions for Death: The Drugging of the Third World (Berkeley: University of California Press, 1982); Abramson, *Overdosed America*.

32   Institute of Medicine, *The Future of Drug Safety*.

33   See Angell, *The Truth*; Abramson, *Overdosed America*; Goozner, *The $800 Million Pill*; Alicia Mundy, *Dispensing with the Truth* (New York: St. Martin's Press, 2001); Petersen, *Our Daily Meds*; H. Waxman, *The Marketing of Vioxx to Physicians* (Washington, DC: United States House of Representatives, Committee on Government Reform, 2005), http://oversight.house.gov/documents/20050505114932-41272.pdf.

34   Abramson, *Overdosed America*, chap. 9; Therapeutics Initiative, "Do Statins Have a Role in Primary Prevention?," *Therapeutics Letter* 48 (Vancouver, Canada: University of British Columbia, April 2003), http://www.ti.ubc.ca/en/TherapeuticsLetters; J. Abramson and J. M. Wright, "Are Lipid-Lowering Guidelines Evidence-Based?" *Lancet* 369 (2007): 168–69.

35   F. R. Curtiss and K. A. Fairman, "Looking for the Outcomes We Love in All the Wrong Places: The Questionable Value of Biomarkers and Investments in Chronic Care Disease Management Interventions," *Journal of Managed Care Pharmacy* 14 (2008): 563–70.

36   C. Starner, J. Shafer, A. Heaton, and P. Gleason, "Rosiglitazone and Polgitazone Utilization from January 2007 Through May 2008 Associated with Four Risk-Warning Events," *Journal of Managed Care Pharmacy* 14 (2008): 523–31.

37   Talcott Parsons, *The Social System* (1951; London: Routledge & Kegan Paul, 1991).

38   Ibid., 450.

39   Ibid., 469.

40   Peter Temin, *Taking Your Medicine: Drug Regulation in the United States* (Cambridge, MA: Harvard University Press, 1980), chap. 9.

41   H. Waxman, *The Marketing of Vioxx to Physicians*; Prescrire International, "15 Years of Monitoring and One Simple Conclusion: Don't Expect Sales Representatives to Help Improve Healthcare Quality," *Prescrire International* 15, no. 84: 1954–59, http://www.prescrire.org/editoriaux/EDIbilanVMEn.pdf.

42   PharmaLive, "National Study by Peoplemetrics Rx Confirms Importance of Emotional Connection Between Pharmaceutical Sales Reps and Physicians," August 11, 2008, http://pharmalive.com/news/index.cfm?articleID=563119&categoryid=9&newsletter=1.

43   A. Pollack, "Amgen Alters Anemia Drug Discounts," *New York Times*, August 28, 2008, C1, C2; R. Abelson, "Quickly Vetted, Treatment is Offered to Cancer Patients," *New York Times*, October 27, 2008, A1, A14. This covert risk to patients occurs in high-priced medical devices as well, such as the radioactive "seeds" implanted tem-

porarily to treat breast cancer, which the FDA approved *without* rigorous testing, on an "experimental" basis. However, any specialist can use them and they do not necessarily tell patients that the benefits and harms have not been evaluated by the FDA. Nor do they mention that the new device generates more than ten times the revenue per day of standard radiation therapy, plus a $20,000 fee for surgery.

44 C. Grassley, "Grassley Questions Increases in Drug Makers Rebates to Physicians Prescribing Anti-Anemia Drugs," U.S. Senate Finance Committee, April 5, 2008, http://finance.senate.gov/press/Gpress/2008/prg040308.pdf; M. Angell, "Drug Companies and Doctors: A Story of Corruption," *New York Review of Books* 56, no. 1 (January 15, 2009).

45 A. Relman, "Separating Continuing Medical Education from Pharmaceutical Marketing," *Journal of American Medical Association* 285 (2001): 2009–12; A. Relman and M. Angell, "America's Other Drug Problem: How the Drug Industry Distorts Medicine and Politics," *The New Republic* 227 (2002): 27–41.

46 M. A. Steinman, L. A. Bero, M-M. Chen, and C. S. Landerfeld, "Narrative Review: The Promotion of Gabapentin: An Analysis of Internal Industry Documents," *Annals of Internal Medicine* 145 (2006): 284–93.

47 D. M. Tran et al., "Physician Communication About the Cost and Acquisition of Newly Prescribed Medications," *American Journal of Managed Care* 12 (2006): 657–64, http://www.ajmc.com/media/pdf/AJMC_06novTarn657to664.pdf.

48 B. Golomb et al., "Physician Response to Patient Reports of Adverse Drug Effects," *Drug Safety* 30 (2007): 669–75. On adverse effects of statins, see G. V. Mann, "Diet-Heart: End of an Era," *New England Journal of Medicine* 297 (1977): 644–50; U. Ravnskov, *The Cholesterol Myths* (Washington, DC: New Trends Publishing, 2000); Brody, *Hooked*; and Abramson, *Overdosed America*.

49 Olson, "Are Novel Drugs More Risky?"; Giezen et al., "Safety-Related Regulatory Actions for Biologicals"; Carpenter et al., "Drug-Review Deadlines and Safety Problems."

50 L. Z. Benet, "Review and Critique of the Institute of Medicine Report, 'The Future of Drug Safety,'" *Clinical Pharmacology & Therapeutics* 82 (2007): 158–61.

51 Carpenter et al., "Drug-Review Deadlines and Safety Problems"; Institute of Medicine, *The Future of Drug Safety*; Olson, "Are Novel Drugs More Risky?"

52 Jacob Hacker, *The Great Risk Shift: The New Economic Insecurity and the Decline of the American Dream*, rev. and exp. ed. (New York: Oxford University Press, 2008).

53 GAO, *FDA Drug Review: Postmarket Risks, 1976–85* (Washington, DC: Government Accountability Office, 1990); S. Okie, "Safety in Numbers—Monitoring Risk in Approved Drugs," *New England Journal of Medicine* 352 (2005): 1173–76.

54 K. E. Lasser et al., "Timing of New Black Box Warnings and Withdrawals for Prescription Medications," *Journal of American Medical Association* 287 (2002): 2215–20.

55 U.S. Office of the Inspector General, *FDA's Review Process for New Drug Applications: a Management Review*, Washington, DC, OEI-01-00590.

56 Abraham, *Science, Politics and the Pharmaceutical Industry*; Goozner, *The $800 Million Pill*; Angell, *The Truth About Drug Companies*; Petersen, *Our Daily Meds*; Jerry Avorn, *Powerful Medicines: The Benefits, Risks and Costs of Prescription Drugs* (New York: Knopf, 2004); Mundy, *Dispensing with the Truth*; Alison Bass, *Side Effects: A Prosecutor, a Whistleblower and Bestselling Antidepressant on Trial* (Chapel Hill, NC: Algonquin Books, 2008); J. Abraham and J. Sheppard, *The Therapeutic Nightmare* (London: Earthscan, 1999).

57 FDA, "Report on the Performance of Drugs and Biologics Firms in Conducting Postmarketing Commitment Studies" (Washington, DC: Federal Register, 2007): 5069-70, http://www.fda.gov/CbER/pstmrkt/pstmrkperfo207.pdf.

58 Institute of Medicine, *Future of Drug Safety*; D. J. Graham, *Testimony of David J. Graham, MD, MPH*, U.S. Senate Finance Committee hearing, November 18, 2004.

59 G. Harris, "Drug Making's Move Abroad Stirs Concerns," *New York Times*, January 20, 2009, D1,D6.

60 Graham, *Testimony*.

61 Waxman, *The Marketing of Vioxx to Physicians*.

62 Prescrire International, "15 Years of Monitoring and One Simple Conclusion: Don't Expect Sales Representatives to Help Improve Healthcare Quality," *Prescrire International* 2006: 154–59; B. Golomb et al., "Physician Response to Patient Reports of Adverse Drug Effects," *Drug Safety* 30 (2007): 669–75; Mundy, *Dispensing with the Truth*; Bass, *Side Effects*.

63 J. S. Ross, K. P. Hill, D. S. Egilman, and H. M. Krumholz, "Guest Authorship and Ghostwriting in Publications Related to Rofecoxib," *Journal of American Medical Association* 299 (2008): 1800–12.

64 Abramson, *Overdosed America*, chap. 3.

65 S. Prakash, "Part 1: Documents Suggest Merck Tried to Censor Vioxx Critics," National Public Radio, June 9, 2005, http://www.npr.org/templates/story/story.php?storyId=4696609; and "Part 2: Did Merck Try to Censor Vioxx Critics?" http://www.npr.org/templates/story/story.php?storyId=4696711&ps=rs. Early knowledge by Merck officers was found by a *Wall Street Journal* investigation as well. See A. Mathews and B. Martinez, "Warning Signs: E-Mails Suggest Merck Knew Vioxx's Dangers at Early Stage," *Wall Street Journal* 2004 (November 1).

66 K. P. Hill, J. S. Ross, D. S. Egilman, and H. M. Krumholz, "The ADVANTAGE

Seeding Trial: A Review Of Internal Documents," *Annals of Internal Medicine* 149 (2008): 251–58.

67 Waxman, *The Marketing of Vioxx to Physicians*; Angell, *The Truth*; Goozner, *The $800 Million Pill*; Mundy, *Dispensing*; Bass, *Side Effects*; Petersen, *Our Daily Meds*.

68 See also Mathews and Martinez, "Warning Signs"; and Petersen, *Our Daily Meds*, 311–15.

69 G. D. Curfman, S. Morrisey, and J. M. Drazen, "Expression of Concern," *New England Journal of Medicine* 343 (2005): 1520–28.

70 Waxman, *The Marketing of Vioxx*.

71 J. Giles, "How Merck Made a Killing," *Prospect Magazine*, November 2008, http://www.prospect-magazine.co.uk/article_details.php?id=10425.

72 At http://www.fda.gov/ohrms/dockets/ac/01/briefing/3677b2_03_med.pdf.

73 Waxman, *The Marketing of Vioxx*.

74 S. Weiss Smith, "Sidelining Safety—the FDA's Inadequate Response to the IOM," *New England Journal of Medicine* 357 (2007): 960–63.

75 S. Pocock, "Innovations in Clinical Trial Design," *NERI News & Views* 2008 (Summer): 1, 19; A. Lakoff, "The Right Patients for the Drug: Managing the Placebo Effect in Antidepressant Trials," *Biosocieties* 2 (2007): 57–71.

76 J. Lenzer, "Contract Research Organizations: Truly Independent Research?" *British Medical Journal* 337 (2008) a1332, http://www.bmj.com/cgi/content/extract/337/aug21_1/a1332.

77 A. Petryna, A. Lakoff, and A. Kleinman, eds., *Global Pharmaceuticals* (Durham, NC: Duke University Press, 2006).

78 Abraham, *Science, Politics and the Pharmaceutical Industry*.

79 A. W. Mathews and B. Martinez, "Warning Signs: E-Mails Suggest Merck Knew Vioxx's Dangers at Early Stage," *Wall Street Journal*, November 1, 2004, A1.

80 On ghost management, see S. Sismondo, "Ghost Management: How Much of the Medical Literature is Shaped Behind the Scenes by The Pharmaceutical Industry?" *PLoS Medicine* 4 (2007): 1429–33; M. A. Steinman, L. A. Bero, Lisa A.Chen, M-M. Landerfeld, and C. Seth, "Narrative Review: The Promotion of Gabapentin: An Analysis of Internal Industry Documents," *Annals of Internal Medicine* 145 (2006): 284–93; Steinman et al., "Characteristics and Impact of Drug Detailing for Gabapentin," *PloS Medicine* 4 (2007): 743–51; B. M. Psaty and W. A. Ray, "FDA Guidance on Off-Label Promotion and the State of the Literature from Sponsors," *Journal of the American Medical Association* 299 (2008): 1949–51. On ghost writing, see Ross et al., "Guest Authorship and Ghostwriting."

81 E. H. Turner, A. M. Matthews, E. Linardatos, R. A. Tell, and R. Rosenthal, "Selective

Publication of Antidepressant Trials and its Influence on Apparent Efficacy," *New England Journal of Medicine* 358 (2008): 252–60.

82 I. Kirsch et al., "Initial Severity and Antidepressant Benefits: A Meta-Analysis of Data Submitted to the Food and Drug Administration," *PLoS Medicine* 5 (2008): e45, http://medicine.plosjournals.org/perlserv/?request=get-document& doi=10.1371/journal.pmed.0050045; D. Healy, *Let Them Eat Prozac: The Unhealthy Relationship Between the Pharmaceutical Industry and Depression* (New York: New York University Press, 2004).

83 A. S. Kesselheim et al., "Clinical Equivalence of Generic and Brand-Name Drugs Used in Cardiovascular Disease," *Journal of the American Medical Association* 300 (2008): 2514–26.

84 M. Procopio, "The Multiple Outcomes Bias in Antidepressants Research," *Medical Hypotheses* 65 (2005): 395–99, 395.

85 D. Wilson, "Investigation Links Wyeth to Articles on Its Drugs," *New York Times*, December 13, 2008, B1.

86 A. J. J. Wood, "Progress and Deficiencies in the Registration of Clinical Trials," *New England Journal of Medicine* 360 (2009):824–30.

87 Wood, "Progress and Deficiencies."

88 Carpenter et al., "Drug-Review Deadlines"; Olson, "Are Novel Drugs More Risky?"; Giezen et al., "Safety-Related Regulatory Actions."

89 Waxman, *The Marketing of Vioxx*.

90 T. H. Maugh, II, "Prescription Drug Injuries and Deaths Reach Record Levels," *Los Angeles Times*, October 23 2008, http://www.latimes.com/features/health/la-sci-drugs23-2008oct23,0,635901.story.

91 M-A. Gagnon and J. Lexchin, "The Cost of Pushing Pills: A New Estimate of Pharmaceutical Promotion Expenditures in the United States," *PLoS Medicine* 8 (2008): 1–5.

92 D. W. Light, "Misleading Congress about Drug Development," *Journal of Health Politics, Policy and Law* 32 (2007): 895–913, http://bioethics.upenn.edu/people/? last=Light&first=Donald.

93 J. M. Donahue, M. Ceveasco, and M. B. Rosenthal, "A Decade of Direct-To-Consumer Advertising of Prescription Drugs," *New England Journal of Medicine* 357 (2007): 673–81.

94 Prescrire International, "Direct-to-Consumer Advertising of Prescription Drugs: Harmful and Difficult to Regulate," *Prescrire International* 17 (2008): 216–17.

95 N. Singer, "Citing Risks, Lawmakers Seek to Curb Drug Commercials," *New York Times*, July 27, 2009, BU1, 6.

96 See T. A. Brennen et al., "Health Industry Practices That Create Conflicts of Inter-
    est," *Journal of the American Medical Association* 295 (2006): 429–33; D. J. Rothman
    et al., "Professional Medical Associations and Their Relationships with Industry,"
    Journal of the American Medical Association 301 (209): 1367–72; Relman, "Separat-
    ing Continuing Medical Education."

97 See the series of news summaries about developments at *Policy and Medicine*, at
    http://www.policymed.com/page/4/.

98 O. O'Donovan, "Corporate Colonization of Health Activism," *International Journal
    of Health Services* 37 (2007); K. Jones, "In Whose Interest? Relationships Between
    Health Consumer Groups and the Pharmaceutical Industry in The UK," *Sociology
    of Health & Illness* 30 (2008): 929–43; Health Action International, *Patients' Groups
    and Industry Funding* (Amsterdam: HAI, 2002).

99 Angell, *The Truth*; Steinman et al., "Narrative Review"; Steinman et al., "Character-
    istics and Impact"; Psaty and Ray, "FDA Guidance on Off-Label"; Wilson, "Investi-
    gation Links Wyeth"; R. S. Stafford, "Regulating Off-Label Drug Use — Rethinking
    the Role of the FDA," *New England Journal of Medicine* 358 (2008): 1427–29.

100 Stafford, "Regulating Off-Label Drug Use"; D. C. Radley, S. N. Finkelstein, and
    R. S. Stafford, "Off-Label Prescribing Among Office-Based Physicians," *Archives
    of Internal Medicine* 66 (2006).

101 Stafford, "Regulating Off-Label Drug Use."

102 GAO, *Prescription Drugs: FDA's Oversight of the Promotion of Drugs for Off-Label
    Uses* (Washington, DC: Government Accountability Office, July 2008).

103 Brownlee, *Overtreated.*

104 Peter Conrad, *The Medicalization of Society* (Baltimore: Johns Hopkins University
    Press, 2007). For an excellent, brief overview of how well people are redefined as
    sick, see the *Seattle Times* series at http://seattletimes.nwsource.com/news/health/
    suddenlysick/. See special issue of *PLoS Medicine*, April 2006, on disease monger-
    ing, such as redefining erectile dysfunction, creating female sexual dysfunction,
    and broadening ADHD and bipolar disorder.

105 N. Singer, "In Push for Cancer Screening, Limited Benefits," *New York Times*, July
    17, 2009, A1, A15.

106 Ray Moynihan and Alan Cassels, *Selling Sickness: How the World's Biggest Phar-
    maceutical Companies Are Turning Us All Into Patients* (New York: Nation Books,
    2005).

107 S. Kelleher and D. Wilson, "Suddenly Sick: What Can Go Wrong When the Drug
    Industry Influences What Constitutes Disease, Who Has It, And How It Should
    Be Treated," *Seattle Times* 2006 (June 26–30), http://seattletimes.nwsource.com/

news/health/suddenlysick/. See also http://www.cspinet.org/new/pdf/integsci_4.24.pdf.

108 P. Campos et al., "The Epidemiology of Overweight and Obesity: Public Health Crisis or Moral Panic?" *International Journal of Epidemiology* 35 (2006): 55–60.

109 Marsa, "Is Your Medicine Making You Sick?" *Ladies Home Journal* July 2008: 88–101 (anniversary issue of the *Ladies Home Journal* publishing its 1908 expose on dangerous drugs).

110 L. Tiefer, "Female Sexual Dysfunction: A Case Study of Disease Mongering and Activist Resistance," *PLoS Medicine* 3 (2006): e178. See entire special issue of *PLoS Medicine* for other examples of disease mongering.

111 G. V. Mann, "Diet-Heart: End of an Era," *New England Journal of Medicine* 297 (1977): 644–50; U. Ravnskov, *The Cholesterol Myths* (Washington, DC: New Trends Publishing, 2000).

112 Reviewed in Curtiss and Fairman, "Looking for the Outcomes We Love."

113 T. Parker-Pope, "Cholesterol Screening is Urged For Young," *New York Times*, July 7, 2008, A11.

114 E. Selvin et al., "Cardiovascular Outcomes in Trials of Oral Diabetes Medications: A Systematic Review," *Archives of Internal Medicine* 281 (2008): 1203–10.

115 A. Horwitz, *Creating Mental Illness* (Chicago: University of Chicago Press, 2001).

116 Abramson, *Overdosed America.*

117 N. Singer, "Medical Papers by Ghostwriters Pushed Therapy," *New York Times*, August 5, 2009.

118 A. Mitchell, D. Kaufman, and L. Rosenberg, *Patterns of Medication Use in the United States: A Report from the Slone Survey, 2006,* http://www.bu.edu/slone/SloneSurvey/AnnualRpt/SloneSurveyWebReport2006.pdf.

119 A. Mitchell, D. Kaufman, and L. Rosenberg, *Patterns of Medication Use.*

120 Kaiser Family Foundation, *Prescription Drug Trends,* September 2008, http://www.kff.org/rxdrugs/upload/3057_07.pdf.

121 D. A. Gorard, "Escalating Polypharmacy," *Qjm.* 99 (November 2006): 797–800.

122 Hacker, *The Great Risk Shift.*

123 Kaiser Family Foundation, *Prescription Drug Trends,* September 2008, http://www.kff.org/rxdrugs/upload/3057_07.pdf.

124 Jacob Hacker, ed., *Health at Risk* (New York: Columbia University Press, 2008).

125 OECD, *Pharmaceutical Pricing Policies in a Global Market* (Paris: Organization for Economic Cooperation and Development, 2008), http://www.oecd.org/document/36/0,3343,en_2649_33929_41000996_1_1_1_37407,00.html.

126 D. M. Tarn et al., "Physician Communication About the Cost of Acquisition of

Newly Prescribed Medications," *American Journal of Managed Care* 12 (2006): 657–64.

127   S. Saul, "In Sour Economy Some Scale Back on Medications," *New York Times*, October 21, 2008..

128   Kaiser Family Foundation, *Prescription Drug Trends*.

129   S. L. Baker, "U.S. National Health Spending, 2006," University of South Carolina School of Public Health, http://hspm.sph.sc.edu/COURSES/Econ/Classes/nhe06/; and Kaiser Family Foundation, *Prescription Drug Trends*.

130   D. W. Light, R. Castellblanch, P. Arrendondo, and D. Socolar, "No Exit and the Organization of Voice in Biotechnology and Pharmaceuticals," *Journal of Health Politics, Policy and Law* 28 (2003): 473–507; J. Oberlander, "Through the Looking Glass: The Politics of the Medicare Prescription Drug, Improvement, and Modernization Act," *Journal of Health Politics, Policy and Law* 32 (2007): 187–219.

131   T. R. Oliver et al., "A Political History of Medicare and Prescription Drug Coverage," *Milbank Quarterly* 82 (2004): 283–354.

132   Oberlander, "Through the Looking Glass."

133   B. Bassler, "Million-Dollar Drugs," *AARP Bulletin* 2008 (Oct): 12–14.

134   G. F. Anderson et al., "Donut Holes and Price Controls," *Health Affairs*, July 21, 2004: W4 396–404; A. B. Frakt et al., "Controlling Prescription Drug Costs," *Journal of Health Politics, Policy and Law* 33 (2008): 1079–1106.

135   D. Light and J. Lexchin, "Foreign Free-Riders and the High Price of American Medicines," *British Medical Journal* 331 (2005): 958–60.

136   D. Light, "Basic Research Funds to Discover Important New Drugs: Who Contributes How Much?" in M. A. Burke, ed., *Monitoring the Financial Flows for Health Research 2005: Behind the Global Numbers* (Geneva: Global Forum for Health Research, 2006), 27–43. On the unused legal mandate to lower prices, see P. S. Arno and M. H. Davis, "Why Don't We Enforce Existing Drug Price Controls? The Unrecognized and Unenforced Reasonable Pricing Requirements Imposed upon Patents Deriving in Whole or in Part from Federally Funded Research," *Tulane Law Review* 75 (2001): 631–92.

CHAPTER TWO

The Food and Drug Administration: Inadequate Protection from Serious Risks

DONALD W. LIGHT

> The FDA is responsible for protecting the public health by assuring the safety, efficacy, and security of human and veterinary drugs.
> — FDA Mission Statement

> There's a total inability of the FDA to carry out its mission.
> — Congressman John Dingell, calling for complete overhaul of FDA, 2008[1]

The U.S. Food and Drug Administration (FDA) is the premier public regulatory body of its kind in the world. No other agency has so many staff and resources or has pioneered so many procedures or techniques to protect public safety and promote the development of better drugs. Yet no other regulatory body has been criticized so extensively for falling down on the job, letting too many risky drugs through, and being too dependent on and close to the industry it is supposed to regulate. When one learns how antiquated its information technology systems are, how difficult it is for the agency to recruit and retain good staff with inadequate compensation packages, and how dependent the agency is on the funding, submissions, and policies of pharmaceutical companies, one realizes that protecting patients from drug risks will require a new level of public demand and strong leadership from the White House.

This chapter provides a short history of how the FDA developed, stage by stage, as public health and safety were threatened by drugs that were mislabeled, sold under misleading claims, or had serious adverse effects on patients. A complementary history could be written about ever-stronger standards to protect individuals from risks posed by improperly prepared and stored foods, additives, and contaminants. An important appendix summarizes how drugs are tested. This history of institution-building reveals the central role of drug companies in both marketing dangerous drugs that led to greater protection and limiting regulatory oversight once passed by Congress.

FOUNDING HISTORY: SELLING DANGEROUS NOSTRUMS TO GULLIBLE CONSUMERS

The development of the FDA and regulations to protect patients from hidden risks and toxic effects arose out of a long history of some (but by no means all) doctors, apothecaries, and manufacturers of medicines making and selling adulterated or dangerous medicines while proclaiming their miraculous powers. Adulterations have been a concern from colonial times, when, in 1638, anyone selling water as a cure for scurvy was punished by whipping.[2] Although "protecting public health" is the central phrase in American and European regulation, safeguarding *individuals* from poisons, toxic ingredients, and misrepresentations they cannot detect has played a central role in developing the FDA and other drug regulatory systems.

At the turn of the twentieth century, the manufacture and marketing of medicines was unregulated, and the contents of the many miracle cures, balms, nostrums, and elixirs were kept secret. The American Medical Association (AMA) stepped into this void and set standards for both manufacturing and marketing with the establishment of the Council on Pharmacy and Chemistry in 1905.[3] Some manufacturers concentrated on selling higher quality medicines to physicians; this formed the basis for modern pharmaceutical companies. Such companies drew on the AMA standards to distinguish themselves from less scrupulous competitors, sharing an interest with doctors of medicine (MDs), who had earlier used licensure laws to set standards that distinguished them from less scientific doctors. Thus, a symbiotic relationship developed between specialists promoting prescription-based drugs and their manufacturers to enhance each other's power and legitimacy that has continued from before the beginning of the era of effective drugs in the 1930s. Drugs sold as higher quality and physician-endorsed also justified higher prices and profits.

As part of a campaign under Theodore Roosevelt to expose dangerous preparations of food and drugs, *The Nation, Collier's,* and *Ladies' Home Journal,* the most popular magazines of the time, published influential articles between 1903 and 1905 on the dangers of widely sold drugs and ingredients.[4] *Collier's* listed the names and addresses of patients who had been killed by them. Scores of bills were proposed to protect an unsuspecting public from hidden risks. Food and drug manufacturers countered vigorously, spending large sums on senators and congressmen to persuade them to bury these bills in committee.

However, the pro-regulatory campaign intensified, and the Pure Food and Drug Act was passed in 1906. It established the principle that the government should protect citizens from risks due to commercial fraud and abuse by outlawing adulterated or mislabeled drugs and foods.[5] This allowed manufacturers to avoid regulation by not listing ingredients except for those required, such as alcohol, opium, cocaine, or marijuana. Testing for safety and claims was not covered; so manufacturers could still claim their drug made people stronger or cured cancer. Congress allocated no funds for enforcement, and federal agents could not prosecute but had to take each case to court. Further, the resulting penalty could not be more than a misdemeanor. In a history of the FDA, Philip Hilts writes that "the meager punishment was a signal heard to the present day.... The secret-ingredient medicine industry, which had fought regulation vigorously, found that the new law was really not very burdensome after all."[6] What reformers should have used as their model, Hilts contends, was the Biologics Control Act of 1902, which required any manufacturer of vaccines to qualify first for a license each year, based on annual inspections. Instead, the law as passed was based on catching violators only after drugs were already being used by millions of people. This proved to be a fatally flawed approach to safety. Labeling aside, the law did little to prevent the exaggerated and even blatantly false claims of advertisements in national periodicals and newspapers that had become the major vehicles for selling medicines.

One case soon after the passage of the Pure Food and Drug Act involved a headache cure containing a painkiller that had previously been found to cause heart attacks, of which millions of bottles were sold. The manufacturer claimed it provided "a most wonderful, certain and harmless relief."[7] A jury found him guilty of mislabeling and fined him $700, which represented less than four one-hundredths of one percent of his profits. He paid and kept selling his headache cure for years, continuing to put consumers at serious risk. In 1910, the FDA took to court the manufacturer of "Johnson's Mild Combination Cancer Treatment," a worthless treatment that claimed to cure cancer, to remove this false claim from the label; the government lost. The judge ruled that claims of effectiveness were not considered mislabeling. In response, Congress passed an amendment that gave the FDA authority to prosecute false claims, but only by taking each case to court to prove the claims to be both false and deliberate. These cases illustrate early, fundamental needs to keep drug companies from deceiving innocent patients, to have enforcement powers, and to exercise consequential sanctions against false or misleading claims. These needs remain partially unfulfilled, as a recent government assessment of the FDA's regulation of off-label promotional materials indicates.[8] Overall, sales of the pharmaceutical industry increased sixfold during the first twenty years under the 1906 act, a testimony to the triumph of marketing over effectiveness, given that few seriously beneficial drugs existed before the first sulfa drug, introduced in 1935.

Under President Franklin Roosevelt and Assistant Secretary of Agriculture Rexford Tugwell, Walter Campbell, the FDA commissioner, proposed legislation to protect patients from the risks of false or exaggerated advertising claims as well as false labeling by requiring that evidence of safety be submitted before approval.[9] The pharmaceutical industry, which emphasized competition and private markets to sort out claims without scientific backing about drugs with undisclosed ingredients, mounted an intense campaign against the bill.[10] Many of the drugs sold to millions depended on false claims, like Lydia Pinkham's wildly popular Vegetable Compound, which contained no vegetables but was 18% alcohol. The bill would have required companies to show that their new drugs were safe *before* they could be sold. Industry indicated that these requirements would decimate drug advertising and retail sales. Government protections from hidden risks and poisons were presented as preventing millions of people from being able to buy their favorite medicines.

Public indifference to this campaign was replaced by widespread support after the Elixir Sulfanilamide disaster in 1937. A drug company had used diethylene glycol (a toxic syrup of antifreeze) to dissolve sulfanilamide into a pleasant-tasting elixir, without testing it or listing it as a new ingredient. Reports soon came in from around the country of patients dying after taking it. FDA inspectors went to the plant and learned that no safety tests had been done on the elixir because none were required, a telling rationale: if not required, there must be no need for tests; but if required, government would be seen as interfering with free enterprise and rapid access to beneficial drugs.

The FDA could not take legal action because deadly drugs were not illegal, only mislabeled drugs. The manufacturer responded to reports of deaths by stating that the elixir had been extensively tested before shipping, contrary to what FDA inspectors found. It said there was no clear proof the elixir had caused the deaths; however, the chemist who had added the antifreeze chemical committed suicide. FDA inspectors fanned out to try to collect all the bottles that had been shipped across the country, but not before 107 people had died. Suddenly, the public realized that the Pure Food and Drug Act did not require testing drugs for safety.

In the wake of the sulfanilamide disaster, Congress passed the 1938 Food, Drug, and Cosmetic Act. It required for the first time in the world that manufacturers test any new drug for safety and report the results before selling it. Although it seemed as if the government would finally be able to keep harmful drugs from patients, the companies could test for safety any way they wanted, without informing patients or keeping records. Further, approval was automatic unless the FDA had proof within sixty days that a new drug was dangerous.[11] Despite these weak provisions, the 1938 law began an era of replacing testimonials, anecdotes, and unfounded claims as "evidence" of safety with scientific testing.

The new law also made safety requirements less stringent if the drugs had to be prescribed by a physician. To ease its regulatory burden, the FDA began to assign most new drugs to the "prescription only" category, thus passing on responsibility for safety to physicians. Historian Peter Temin believes this change represented a loss in consumer sovereignty and a new layer of regulatory gatekeeping by licensed physicians.[12] But the industry saw the advantages of having to market only to physicians rather than to the entire nation and vigorously promoted the institutional construction of "prescription drugs" as a prevalent legal and commercial category.

Companies hired thousands of sales reps to visit doctors personally and emphasize the benefits of each new drug. They created catchy names to replace that of the active ingredient and often used different names in different countries. This made protecting patients from safety more difficult, especially in Europe and Latin America, because a dangerous drug like thalidomide was marketed under different names in different countries so it did not have a single, readily identifiable name. Heavy marketing to the profession led to using brand names for medical training, educational materials, and the entire professional culture, in contrast to Great Britain, where the entire professional culture uses generic names, even for new drugs.

Company marketing directly to doctors and advertising revenues of the AMA journals grew rapidly, as did the art of professional persuasion by sales representatives, who developed personal friendships, left free samples of new products, and spent liberally on doctors. It takes 10–12% of revenues to sell products with no particular feature, like gum, candy, or soda; so one would expect much less would be needed to market products to professionals who know their real benefits.[13] Yet by the 1960s, the pharmaceutical industry was spending 20–24% of revenues to market to physicians, only one five-hundreth of the population that needs to be reached for gum or soda. Companies spent about four times more on selling than on doing research, yet created thousands of new drugs. Dr. Harry Dowling, an officer of the AMA, wrote, "In many fields there are too many drugs that differ so little that they are practically the same. Instead of 24 antihistaminic drugs, we would be better off with five or six and still have enough for vigorous competition. And there are hundreds of mixtures of drugs that have no excuse for being."[14] He estimated that each year 200 to 400 new drugs were launched, only three of which offered new benefits. The director of promotion for Parke-Davis testified in 1959 that the industry turned out 3,790,908,000 pages of journal advertisements and made 741,213,700 direct mail pieces, while its drug reps paid eighteen to twenty million visits to physicians and pharmacists a year, plying them with free samples and favors.[15] By the 1960s, four-fifths of all medicines were prescribed by physicians who received most of their information about new drugs from sales reps, not from the FDA or independent sources.[16] These patterns of flooding the market with drugs that offer few new benefits and surrounding physicians with promotional information have characterized the relationship between the pharmaceutical industry and society to this day.

STREPTOMYCIN

The institutional challenges of safeguarding the public from unsuspected risks are illustrated by the case of Streptomycin, the first antibiotic to successfully treat tuberculosis. Although the drug saved thousands of lives, it had serious and sometimes fatal side effects; yet Parke-Davis promoted it as a miracle drug for many other uses where benefits to offset harms were unclear. When adverse reactions were first reported to the company, it ignored or denied them and continued to market the drug aggressively in a pattern very similar to Merck's response fifty years later to reports of cardiovascular trauma from taking Vioxx.[17] Sales catapulted Parke-Davis from minor to major status among the world's largest pharmaceutical companies.

Reports of severe reactions and death came in daily to the FDA, but at that time it had no systematic safety monitoring system to collect and evaluate adverse event reports. Finally, in 1952, the FDA pressured Parke-Davis to add a few lines of fine print about the side effects and to send out a letter to all physicians. As is typical of company letters required by the FDA, it understated the risk by saying there had been a few reports of blood problems but they were unproven and extremely rare.[18]

Outside the United States, the company continued to promote Streptomycin with no warnings. More reports came in of patients dying, and the FDA pressed for the company to take further action. Parke-Davis kept minimizing the evidence and urging doctors to prescribe it "for the treatment of any disease as they see fit." Deaths mounted, lawsuits proliferated, and independent studies affirmed the dangerousness of the drug; but doctors kept prescribing it until the company stopped marketing it because it went off patent. Hilts concludes, "The FDA again and again was unable to bring itself to restrict the use of the drug."[19] Thus as the modern pharmaceutical industry grew after World War II, it infused the FDA with a pro-industry culture that undermined the agency's ability to protect patients from unsuspected risks.

This case contains many of the elements of the thalidomide disaster but ten years earlier: a drug with serious side effects marketed for several uses of unproven benefit that exposed millions to its risks, repeated denials that patients were being harmed, and continued marketing as more patients were harmed.

A DRUG CRISIS AND THE MODERN FDA

The ambitious populist Senator Estes Kefauver held hearings in the late 1950s highlighting the greed of several industries that exploited the common man, including the drug industry. Testimony by industry leaders and critics at his hearings generated headline after headline about how customers were charged up to 1800% more than cost, how companies spent much more on marketing than they did on research to develop better drugs, how they underplayed the seriousness of toxic side effects, and how many new drugs were known by companies to have no benefit but could be successfully marketed.[20] The former medical director of Squibb testified that for half of all new drugs, "it is clear while they are on the drawing board that they promise no utility; they promise sales."[21] The FDA had no authority to regulate the behavior of physicians or prices. Kefauver wanted the FDA to give generics memorable names rather than names that were difficult to pronounce or remember. FDA officials had no interest. He recommended that each drug company be licensed, subject to renewal after review. FDA officials opposed the idea. The chief of the antibiotics division was found to have received $287,000 (at least $2.2 million in today's dollars) from companies who advised him how to decide issues. A medical officer at the FDA said officers of companies had more influence with FDA officials than its own medical staff, a pattern found in later decades as well. An expert in pharmacology said drugs were approved without rigorous testing, resulting in patients being damaged and twenty-four drugs being recalled.[22]

Kefauver asked questions: Why does the FDA itself not supply doctors with objective, scientific information on new drugs? Why does the FDA not prohibit the proliferation of thousands of Madison Avenue brand names? Why does the FDA itself not send out warning letters to physicians rather than having companies write them? And why does the FDA not concern itself with pricing and value rather than allowing patients to be charged exorbitant prices for medicines their doctors tell them they need? Through such questioning Kefauver outlined what good government could do to minimize bodily and financial risk to patients. Industry leaders responded as they have ever since, that such actions would keep patients from benefiting from innovations and would thus leave untreated patients to suffer or die.

Kefauver's strong reform bill gave the FDA oversight of systematic testing for efficacy and safety before approval. The AMA, by then so dependent on pharmaceutical revenues for advertisements and sponsorships that it had closed down its program to test and approve drugs in the 1950s, joined the industry in opposing it.[23] Senior officials and pharmaceutical leaders again removed oversight of advertising and weakened requirements to prove efficacy. But people's trust in the pharmaceutical industry had declined. Kefauver had shown the industry could not be trusted to regulate the safety of its own products and a stronger FDA was needed to protect patients from risks.

THALIDOMIDE — CONCERN FOR SAFETY PREVENTS DISASTER

In the middle of these negotiations, the thalidomide disaster hit the papers. In Germany, the Grünenthal pharmaceutical company had discovered that thalidomide had a calming effect in lab rats and paid doctors to "test" it by prescribing it to their patients—an example of fusing marketing with testing.[24] Their anecdotal reports varied, from glowing success to concern about dangerous side effects. The company then used the glowing reports to mass-market thalidomide in Europe and Africa. When doctors wrote in about nerve-based side effects, court records later showed, the company wrote back expressing surprise, saying it was the first time they had heard of it, just as Parke-Davis and others had done before.[25]

Two American pharmaceutical companies tested it, found it to have toxic side effects, and decided not to market it; but a subsidiary of Vicks, maker of VapoRub and cough drops, signed on. Vicks and Grünenthal decided that marketing thalidomide to women for reducing nausea during early pregnancy would generate additional sales, though no clinical trial was done to test this off-label use. Instead of testing thalidomide in pregnant women, they felt it would be more effective to have a physician write an article in the *Journal of Obstetrics and Gynecology* testifying that it worked well in pregnancy. An obstetrician, the friend of a Vicks executive, agreed to write the article and claim that thalidomide had been tested, though court records later showed he did not keep records of how many pills he dispensed to whom.[26] He let the company's medical director write the article for him, an early example of a ghostwritten journal article on the alleged safety and efficacy of a new drug. To further market it, Vicks sent half a million pills to more than twelve hundred doctors, many at teaching hospitals, to try out as a "pre-approval trial." Neither the company nor most of the physicians kept records of which patients took the drug or its effects.

A new FDA medical officer, Frances Kelsey, had been given the thalidomide application as her first case. It seemed to be a simple sedative already widely used in Europe and Africa. Well trained in research, she did not like the glowing testimonials being used as "evidence" of safety and asked for better data. Neither company had tested the drug; it seemed much safer than barbiturates because no one was said to have reported side effects. Kelsey refused to approve it until the companies produced more evidence that it was safe. Company executives went over her head to pressure the FDA into approving the drug for the U.S. market. They provided more "evidence." The German company testified there were only thirty-four reported cases of adverse events; later investigations found they had received more than four hundred reports at the time. The American company sent distinguished physicians to testify how beneficial thalidomide was.

Meantime, the German company estimated that by the fall of 1961 at least four thousand babies had been born with "seal limbs," no bowel opening, no ear openings, or segmented intestines. It started quietly settling lawsuits in Europe, where it dropped "non-toxic" from its marketing materials, but it kept marketing thalidomide in Africa as "completely harmless."[27] Finally, one German doctor spoke out, causing a furor in the press. The company pulled thalidomide off the market, blaming a sensationalist press rather than itself for putting patients at risk. Neither company ever admitted there was a problem with the drug, and none of this information was made public to American patients. Frances Kelsey was still holding out against pressure from her superiors to approve thalidomide so that American women could benefit from its innovative features.

When the FDA commissioner, George P. Larrick, learned of the widespread birth defects in Europe, he took no action to round up the pills that had been sent out to thousands of doctors as a "trial" but instead asked the American company what it wanted to do.[28] Kelsey insisted that FDA officers get a list of all the doctors from the company, but it had none. While these internal struggles about how the FDA should respond were taking place, Morton Mintz of the *Washington Post* broke the story: "Heroine of FDA Keeps Bad Drug Off Market."[29] Overnight, Kelsey went from being the obstinate medical reviewer keeping American mothers from enjoying the benefits of a drug widely used in Europe to being a model of the FDA's scientific ability and ethical mandate to protect American mothers and their babies from a tragic fate. Approved as a sleeping pill in forty-two countries, thalidomide caused an estimated ten thousand babies to be born with birth defects.

The Kefauver-Harris Amendment to the 1938 law that was passed in 1962 required the evaluation of old drugs, proof of effectiveness and safety for all new drugs *prior* to approval, disclosure of contraindications on their labels, overview of advertising, and reporting of all adverse effects made known to companies. Definitions of effectiveness and safety, according to Temin, were unclear and meant only what experts said they meant.[30] The FDA gained new powers to withdraw approved drugs if its experts considered them unsafe or lacking evidence of effectiveness. The subsequent review of old drugs demonstrated how extensively the risks of harm to patients had been privatized by companies in the past. About half were found not to be effective, evidence that companies devoted most of their efforts to developing clinically ineffective new drugs and then marketing them successfully as effective. While hundreds of prescription drugs were removed from use, hundreds more ineffective drugs stayed on and continued to be prescribed by physicians.[31]

For decades, the old patent medicine industry and the new research-based pharmaceutical industry had relied on testimonials and informal trials, with no controls, to test new drugs. When a drug was questioned, they still pressured FDA medical reviewers and their superiors for approval. James Goddard, the first person from outside the industry to be named commissioner of the FDA (in 1963), was so shocked at the amateur, unprofessional, and dishonest submissions by companies of the tests on their most promising new drugs that he ordered FDA staff not to waste their time and immediately send back any such applications for resubmission.[32] Patients should not have to bear the risks of poorly tested drugs, he said.

Goddard brought in a new breed of well-trained research physicians and scientists to enable the FDA to carry out its mandates objectively and free of politics. Companies objected to clinical trials and protested that only "medical experience" could tell whether a drug worked and physicians should be the judges. This conflict underscored two different approaches to reliable knowledge and the view of the new FDA that doctors' clinical experiences can never be reliable because they lack the perspective of systematic sampling and controls to validate their personal observations with their patients. The U.S. Supreme Court supported this view in its interpretation of the act. Yet the current system relies heavily on doctors' individual clinical experience once a drug is approved, even though it is acknowledged that the safety of new drugs is not well known until they have been used for a while. In other words, the current system at its best permits a significant amount of risk to be shifted to patients and their doctors, as reflected in the proliferation of toxic side effects described in Chapter 1.

ANTI-REGULATORY BACKLASH

With the election of Richard Nixon in 1968, a sustained campaign began to place conservative Republicans within regulatory agencies. Nixon kept count of the number of Republicans and Democrats in the FDA and vowed to take "political control."[33] Six career officers with almost seventy years of combined FDA experience were transferred without cause or explanation to makeshift jobs. Eleven more reviewers known for their emphasis on patient safety later received abrupt transfers.

In August 1974, Senator Edward Kennedy organized a hearing about these actions, unannounced so that Nixon's FDA leader could not take preemptive action. The transferred officers testified about the double standard of being supported when they recommended approval but overruled when they recommended that new drugs not be approved because they posed serious risks to patients.[34] They experienced harassment and being reassigned to marginal tasks. Evidence was found that FDA management had a policy to "neutralize" reviewing officers who were not "cooperative" with companies. These patterns persist in studies of review officers and industry influence. The net effect, of course, is to silence scientific debate and pass on risks of serious side effects to patients, rather than protecting them.

Starting in the mid 1970s, the pharmaceutical industry sponsored economists and conferences emphasizing how the heightened standards of safety and efficacy since the 1962 amendment were cutting into profits, reducing companies' ability to fund research, and keeping American patients from enjoying the benefits of new drugs that were approved more quickly abroad.[35] Millions of patients were dying, they claimed, because of the lag between when drugs were approved in the United Kingdom and in the United States.[36] These "drug-lag" studies, however, assume that all new drugs are better and therefore any delay harms patients, while in fact the FDA's research showed that only one in every nine new drugs in the 1960s and 1970s provided superior therapeutic benefits to existing ones.[37] From 1981 to 2006, this record improved a little to one in every seven new drugs offering substantial therapeutic advantages.[38] Delayed use of most equivalent drugs reduces risk of harm to patients, which is why the Health Research Group recommends waiting seven years before taking a new drug unless there is no substitute and a patient needs it. A study by the Group found that after higher standards for testing and safety were put in place in 1962, the United States had one-third as many drugs pulled from the market because of their toxic side effects as did France, Germany, and the United Kingdom.[39]

In 1980, the General Accounting Office issued a detailed report on the "lengthy process that delays the availability of important new drugs."[40] It found, in fact, that companies themselves caused many of the delays by not providing vital information to reviewers, by turning their attention to other drugs, by mishandling their applications, and by not responding to legitimate questions from FDA reviewers. The severe lack of staff at the FDA also caused delays as the reviewers got pulled away to do other tasks and handle unexpected safety problems.

The "crisis of overregulation" never calculated the benefits of FDA reviews to patients and to industry in *not* approving dangerous drugs. The costs of harm from weaker regulation were not estimated either.

Budget cuts of the FDA started under President Carter. President Reagan issued Executive Order 12291 and took over control of all regulations from Congress. Anti-regulation leaders found myriad ways to reduce safety inspections as they did across the board in "the great risk shift" to individuals in the name of greater choice.[41] Reagan's Office of Management and Budget drew up a list of the "terrible twenty" regulations for classifying hazardous waste and pollutants and for giving patients more information about drugs in package inserts. Arthur Hayes, a highly paid consultant to drug companies, was selected as commissioner of the FDA and immediately turned to cancelling the new program to provide information directly to patients about the drugs they were taking, a program the pharmaceutical industry fiercely opposed. FDA staff was cut from 7,960 in 1978 to 6,960 in 1987 at the same time that the FDA was assigned more tasks in overseeing one-fifth of the U.S. economy. Seizures and prosecutions dropped from 500 to 173, leaving the industry to regulate itself. It responded by decreasing its voluntary actions by 800 a year.[42] This recent history makes clear again that privatizing risk does not mean that industry will protect patients by policing itself.

Despite the cuts in staff and resources, and in response to the anti-regulation campaign, the FDA worked hard during the 1980s to speed up reviews by helping companies complete their applications properly, by working with company researchers to get quicker responses to questions or missing data, and by tightening the review process. One obstacle was the continued lack of professional submissions by companies that Goddard had found in the early 1960s. A survey of FDA reviewers in the mid 1990s published in *Pharmaceutical Executive* reported that a third of drug applications "were essentially unreadable and could not even be considered."[43] The reviewers considered only 30% to be good and 7% excellent.[44]

Working with companies and improving review procedures paid off. The average time for standard reviews dropped from thirty-three months in 1987 to nineteen months in 1992, then to sixteen months by 1994. Nevertheless, Representative Newt Gingrich launched a campaign through his Progress and Freedom Foundation to eliminate the FDA. The Washington Legal Foundation published ads claiming that delays in approval had killed at least twenty-five hundred kidney cancer patients who could not get Interleukin-2 while the FDA reviewed the drug and caused fourteen thousand patients to have heart attacks because they could not benefit from the CardioPump during its two-year review.[45] The facts did not support these allegations, and industry leaders became worried that the vitriolic attack could kill the goose (the FDA) that was laying the golden eggs, FDA-approved drugs. FDA procedures could hardly have been regarded as hostile to the industry. On the contrary, as described in Chapter 1, they let through a substantial number of drugs that had serious risks. Thomas Moore of George Washington University estimated that lifetime chances of severe injury from auto accidents were two in one hundred but twenty-six in one hundred from prescription drugs.[46] Hearings in May 1996 led to the campaign being discredited and the bill dying in committee, but they highlighted the business view that the less regulation the better so that new products can get on the market quickly.[47] The way to maximize product availability is not to regulate at all; let companies develop what drugs they want, test them as they see best, and sell them. This view is put forward by industry-friendly authors and journalists to this day, without consideration that uncertainty surrounds the risks of all new drugs and only a few provide offsetting advantages.[48]

INDUSTRY FUNDS ITS REGULATOR

The FDA became so demoralized and overburdened that the industry itself became concerned lest the benefits of having their products approved by a respected agency become compromised.[49] It created an FDA advocacy council to find ways to improve regulatory operations. The solution that emerged was a "user fee" system: companies would pay for each new drug application, which would provide much-needed money to hire more than two hundred new reviewers. The Prescription Drug User Fee Act (PDUFA) became law in 1992.

The industry, in return for paying large fees to substitute for Congress adequately funding the FDA, required in 1992 (PDUFA I) that 90% of reviews for all priority drugs and supplements be completed in less than six months and those for standard drugs and supplements in less than twelve months. It also required that all fees go to reviewing new drugs for approval and "specifically prohibited the use of fees for any postmarketing drug safety activities."[50] Unlike the fixed-fee schedule

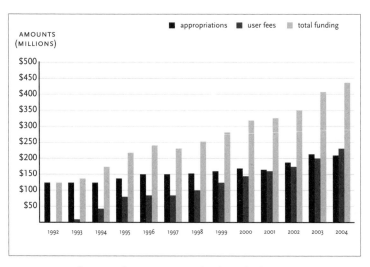

Figure 2.1   Rise of corporate fees as proportion of total FDA funding

[Source: Institute of Medicine, Committee on the Assessment of the US Drug Safety System, *The Future of Drug Safety: Promoting and Protecting the Health of the Public* (Washington, DC: National Academies Press, 2007), 194]

used in Europe, the industry set up PDUFA so that it could renegotiate further conditions in return for its fees every five years. For the 1998–2002 continuation (PDUFA II), the pharmaceutical industry accelerated reviews of standard products to 90% in ten months and added several new requirements that FDA staff respond more quickly and fully to industry requests for meetings and resolving disputes.[51] Corporate fees have gone from about one-tenth of total FDA funding to more than half (figure 2.1).[52]

The accelerated reviews — often based on short-term surrogate or substitute changes instead of true clinical improvement — combined with mass-marketing of these new medications for uses approved and unapproved, created a dangerous situation.[53] An estimated twenty million or more Americans were exposed to drugs approved under PDUFA I that were then withdrawn soon after for their severe adverse effects. Warnings were added to many others.

A case in point was the diabetes drug Rezulin. After the FDA reviewer Dr. John Gueriguian pointed out that it offered no substantial advantages over the other eight diabetes drugs already on the market but showed signs of liver toxicity, Warner-Lambert officers went over his head to FDA officials and pressured them to remove him from the case, just as companies have done so many times before, including the attempt to remove Frances Kelsey from the thalidomide case. Time and again, FDA reviewers and scientists carry out rigorous, scientific assessments but are overruled or barred or removed if they believe that safety risks are enough to rule out drug approval. As reports of deaths began to come in, the British Medicines Control Agency banned Rezulin. The FDA considered one kind of warning, negotiating a series of labeling changes and letters to doctors asking for increasingly more liver monitoring—which were largely ignored as the death toll mounted over the next year and a half.[54] Only after Warner-Lambert developed a second drug in the class that was approved and found not to cause liver damage did the company stop marketing Rezulin. Thus both the review before approval and response to serious harm afterward were compromised by not having a regulatory body not subject to industry influence. The professionals were there, capable and dedicated, but the upper echelons did not support their work.

In response to growing criticism and the rash of new drugs doing serious damage to patients, the FDA organized a task force; it "identified process, resource, and statutory constraints on [the] FDA's ability to identify adverse events."[55] Finally, in the 2002 renewal for 2003–2007 (PDUFA III), "limited funds were allocated for limited safety activities."[56] Then the Vioxx disaster occurred and set off major congressional hearings as well as a full-press review by the Institute of Medicine (IOM) that resulted in major recommendations for organizational, legal, and cultural changes.[57]

The IOM concluded that the "FDA does not have adequate resources or procedures for translating preapproval safety signals [evidence of harm to patients] into effective postmarketing studies, for monitoring and ascertaining the safety of new marketed drugs, for responding promptly to the safety problems that are discovered after marketing approval, and for quickly and effectively communicating appropriate risk information to the public."[58] In other words, the FDA was not capable of protecting patients from harmful risks in the drugs they take. This conclusion is supported by key themes and documentation in Chapter 1. Some reports go further. Two investigative reporters, for example, wrote a three-part series in 2003 describing the extent of off-label or unauthor-ized use that makes the forty-year effort to assure that drugs are safe and effective irrelevant.[59] Byron Richards describes how the Bush administra-tion appointed industry advocates to key FDA positions so that acceler-ated reviews could be combined with blocking patients from suing for damages from resulting injuries.[60]

The industry-required speed-up has resulted in substantially more risk for patients from drugs approved in the last two months before the tightened deadlines than drugs approved earlier, presumably because there were more concerns about them but not enough time to resolve them. According to a study at Harvard, deadline-crunch approvals have resulted in drugs being put on the market that are three times more likely to result in toxic effects leading to severe, black-boxed warnings because of serious harms and being pulled from the market altogether, compared to drugs that the FDA had no trouble approving within the time allotted.[61]

PARTIAL STRENGTHENING OF SAFETY PROTECTION

Questions about the ability of the FDA to ensure the safety of approved medicines[62] led Congress to pass in 2007 an historic set of changes to strengthen protection in the Food and Drug Administration Amend-ments Act (FDAAA), which gave the agency new regulatory power, more money, and safety-related mandates.[63] The IOM drug safety panel mem-bers noted that Congress "responded in full" to the recommendations of their committee but were more critical of the FDA's own response that preceded FDAAA.[64]

The new act requires the FDA to develop rigorous safety measures and to evaluate at regular intervals the risk minimization action plans of companies. It provides the authority to require post-market studies, label changes, and restrictions on distribution when deemed necessary, with substantial penalties. A safety officer is assigned to each of the seventeen groups that evaluate new drug applications. A national sentinel system is being developed that will combine patient data from a number of large health systems to identify and evaluate risks and harms through analy-sis of clinical data. This is part of a larger set of activities to implement the Institute of Medicine's lifecycle approach to drug safety—testing for safety not just before approval but through each phase of a drug's life.[65]

Despite the agency's new safety initiatives, "Major obstacles remain. They include inadequate resources, the complexity of the science, . . . a dysfunctional organizational culture, problems with credibility and public trust, and the lack of adequate communication about and limited public awareness of drug risks and benefits."[66] The FDA has "computer systems so old that repairmen must be called out of retirement to fix them."[67] It has vital information on databases that are incompatible with each other. It has too few inspectors to monitor the quality of active ingredients as well as the fillers, binders, coatings, and syrups used in drugs; four-fifths of these are imported, mostly from uninspected chemical plants throughout Asia.

Although the "culture of safety" that the IOM emphasized has begun to develop, counterbalancing the substantial gains, "the very structure of the FDA marginalizes safety."[68] Regulatory authority to take action when patients experience toxic side effects still rests with the division that approved the drug. Decisions on safety-related labeling changes, warnings, and even the design and evaluation of epidemiological safety and risk management studies can still be done without the input of epidemiology safety specialists, who serve on a consultancy basis, only when called upon. Even when safety officers are called in, the tug-of-war between the public health perspective—on managing risks and benefits across all users—and the more narrow medical perspective of treating an individual patient with the drug results in conflicting professional opinions. Internal disagreements are often quashed or ignored, the most egregious playing out on the front pages of leading newspapers and in congressional testimony, as the agency struggles to present a unified front amid scientific uncertainty.

The FDA has quickly moved into the business of meeting its new statutory requirements. The scale of change, including the development of completely new systems and processes, is daunting, and the FDA is now hiring hundreds of new scientists and inspectors. Will the FDA be able to hire the highly specialized workforce that it needs to do the job? Its science infrastructure is dated and weak, victim of years of underfunding; the FDA science board has only half the funding it needs.[69] Hiring and retaining good people is frustrated by salaries that are about half those in industry and by the weakening of the once-legendary federal pension system. This, plus strict rules against stock ownership among FDA employees, almost assures that the flow of well-trained regulatory scientists is in just one direction—from FDA to industry. Fully funding the FDA would cost about four cents per person per day, or $4.38 billion.[70]

In 2008, two congressional leaders concluded that the extensive reforms of 2007 were not enough. Senator Charles Grassley and Representative John Dingell called for restructuring the FDA to "build a much taller wall between the agency and the industry it regulates."[71] The FDA needs the power to recall drugs and impose stiff fines, and new leadership must "fix the culture." Safety reviewers should have "complete autonomy," Senator Grassley said. Senator Arlen Specter called the FDA "a joke." A staunch defender of the FDA, Peter Barton Hutt no longer will defend it: "This is a fundamentally broken agency," he told the *New York Times*.[72] A score of congressional investigations into specific issues have been started, such as paying physicians for each injection of powerful drugs, industry influence on professional education, and paying generic manufacturers not to put a drug on the market.

It would be fair to say the picture is mixed. On one hand, the FDA has become much more serious about protecting patients from risks. It has issued blanket warnings, for example, against whole classes of drugs for small children, and it has finally taken seriously evidence that the whole class of antidepressants known as SSRI drugs, based on surrogate end points, are not very effective and have serious side effects. It has moved swiftly when poisonous foods are discovered, and it has become much more worried about the safety of active ingredients imported from China and elsewhere that go into most drugs Americans take. On the other hand, drug safety was not given its own organizational division or the kinds of powers that leading experts and physicians said were necessary to protect patients from serious risks. Up-against-the-deadline approvals still continue, when the rules could be amended to allow more time for FDA reviewers when they need it to complete a good assessment of the one drug in every three to four that has unresolved concerns. Most important, Congress has not yet fully funded the FDA, so it remains the guardian against hidden risks funded by the industry it monitors. Full funding for independent safety regulation would be a bargain, given that the FDA is the public's guardian for one-fifth of the economy, the fifth that we take into our bloodstreams.

Today's drug approval process is highly scripted, with volumes of regulatory documents to guide product testing and contents of the new drug application and a schedule for meetings and regulatory decisions. FDA approval to market a new prescription medication requires that companies conduct extensive studies in animals and in humans, which takes years and costs millions of dollars. Sponsors must provide the FDA with "substantial evidence" of the drug's effectiveness from well-controlled clinical trials and of the drug's safety relative to the benefits that can be derived when prescribed for the intended or labeled condition(s).[73]

The process begins with a sponsor (usually a pharmaceutical company) submitting an Investigational New Drug (IND) application with proposed trial designs; a review team from one of seventeen disease- or treatment-based divisions of the Office of New Drugs reviews the application within thirty days to see if there are safety concerns.[74] Phase 1 trials test different doses in a small number of healthy subjects to measure safety and tolerability. In Phase 2, companies carry out clinical investigations in 40–400 patients to administer different doses in order to measure efficacy, safety, and tolerability (in ways described in Chapter 1 to maximize evidence of effectiveness and minimize evidence of toxic side effects). Phase 3 trials usually involve about 400–2,000 patients each, randomly assigned to take the new study drug or a placebo, typically without the patients knowing which they are using, to test more formally for efficacy, safety, and tolerability.

It is commonly said that drug development takes twelve to fifteen years. However, preclinical development usually takes two to three years and is relatively inexpensive. The average time for trials has declined in recent years from under six years to less than three, and FDA review is now six to ten months.[75] Thus drug development time is six to seven years, while the time it takes to discover a new drug has never been documented but appears to vary from a few months (for example, the discovery of Viagra as a side effect of a heart drug) to years of research by multiple teams as they run into dead ends and false discoveries before finally identifying an active ingredient that works.[76] Most basic research and funding of discovery is funded by taxpayers.[77] To say that it takes twelve to fifteen years to develop a drug is therefore inaccurate, and no verifiable data support this industry estimate. Costs are commonly estimated to be $1–2 billion, based on unverified industry data, often analyzed by industry-supported economists.[78] Independent data, such as companies' audited tax returns and FDA data on trial sizes, suggest that median net corporate costs are about one-tenth these estimates.[79] Trials are shortest and corporate costs are lowest for cancer and AIDS drugs, yet they are priced the highest.[80] About eight to nine out of every ten drugs that enter clinical trials are withdrawn by the company, usually because test results or commercial potential are considered insufficient.

When trials are completed, a final New Drug Application (NDA) is submitted, often in a rolling fashion involving twenty-four to seventy partial submissions containing two hundred thousand pages of material.[81] The FDA review team first determines if elements are missing and asks for them. Once the application is determined by the FDA to be complete, final review begins. This drug-review system "inevitably puts drugs on the market when safety information is incomplete,"[82] not just for rare side effects but also for those which occur under common but untested conditions, such as long-term usage or interactions with foods or other drugs. Although NDAs often have evidence of a therapeutic benefit for acute diseases, for chronic conditions, benefits are typically based on surrogate or substitute endpoints and a research model that may or may not benefit hard clinical endpoints.[83] Thus, as part of approving a drug, the FDA often outlines Phase 4 postapproval trials or studies to gather further information on safety and effectiveness. Most, however, are not started, and few are completed. An FDA analysis in 2006 found that companies had completed only 11% of 1,259 agreed-on studies.[84] These studies would have provided valuable information about the risks passed on to patients. On the other hand, companies conduct many new studies to gather data supporting wider, off-label uses and marketing efforts for approved drugs.

Although the approval decision is often couched in terms of weighing a drug's benefits against its adverse side effects, or calculating a "risk-benefit ratio," the approval decision-making process is no mathematical exercise. There are standard methods for quantifying or comparing risks and benefits and no scale that could allow comparison between drugs. The risk-benefit ratio is a qualitative judgment made by experts based on available data that is largely generated and presented by the sponsoring company.

An adverse event that occurs rarely, in just one person out of every one thousand persons using a medication, will result in about five hundred events among one-half million people taking the drug, or ten thousand adverse events for every ten million patients taking a drug. For example, commonly used nonsteroidal anti-inflammatory drugs (NSAIDS), which include aspirin and acetaminophen, cause gastrointestinal (GI) bleeding in approximately 7.3 and 13 per 1,000, respectively, among persons with osteoarthritis and rheumatoid arthritis.[85] Although the risk seems small, half of the estimated 200,000–400,000 annual hospitalizations for GI bleeding involve NSAIDS. An estimated 16,500 NSAID-related deaths occur annually just among patients with rheumatoid arthritis or osteoarthritis.[86]

Benefits are multidimensional and may occur quickly (e.g., symptom relief) or many years in the future (e.g., preventing disease or future disability). Benefits need to be considered in terms of the type of disease being treated, the impact of the active ingredient on the disease, how the disease progresses without treatment (its natural history), and alternative treatments already on the market. Risks are typically considered in terms of frequency, severity, preventability, and predictability. For cancer treatments a high rate of toxicity is often an acceptable trade-off against a chance of longer survival. Conversely, for drugs that offer limited benefits, such as relief of headache or cold symptoms, less risk is tolerated by reviewers. Somewhere in between are drugs for which risks may be acceptable among a unique group of patients, under specific circumstances (e.g., failure of all other treatment options), or where risk can be reduced, avoided, or prevented with intervention. These trade-offs are illustrated in figure 2.2. In such cases, the FDA may require some type of risk management program, which can range from patient education (with or without a required paper trail) to required, continuous monitoring of physiologic measures to determine if the medication can be taken by the patient.

In some situations, particularly when evaluating drugs for imminently life-threatening conditions, treatments for rare conditions, and perhaps in some circumstances for patients who have exhausted all approved treatment options, the current bar may be appropriate. For drugs for common chronic conditions, such as hypertension, diabetes, pain, and obesity, with the potential to be quickly prescribed to large

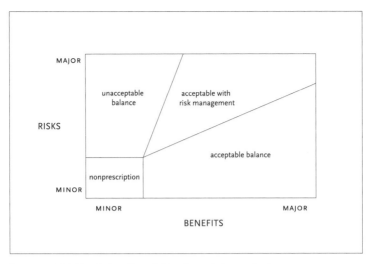

Figure 2.2   Weighing the benefits and risks of prescription medications

[Source: CIOMS IV (1998), adapted in S. R. Weiss, "Approaches to Quantifying the Risk/Benefit Balance"

(FDA visiting lecture, Rockville, Maryland, January 11, 2005)]

numbers of people upon approval, the current bar is too low to prevent widespread adverse effects from occurring.[87] It puts all decision making where it has traditionally resided—with the physician (prescriber) and the patient. However, because preapproval studies are not designed to evaluate risks of long-term usage nor typically overall survival, vital information that is needed to make a truly informed decision is often unavailable or nonexistent sometimes years after approval.

Historically, the FDA has applied a perspective that can lead to millions of patients being exposed to unsuspected risks when making benefit-risk evaluations. Reviewers ask, "Are there patients whom physicians might conceivably see in their clinical practice, for whom the benefits would outweigh the risks?" Many times the answer is yes: some physicians have some patients who might benefit. But this permissive criterion does not consider how an approved drug is then marketed to as many physicians as possible for them to prescribe it for as many patients as possible—the risk proliferation syndrome (see Chapter 1).

NOTES

1   Alicia Mundy, "Grassley, Dingell Lead Calls for Overhauling FDA," *Wall Street Journal*, July 30, 2008.

2   Philip J. Hilts, *Protecting America's Health: The FDA, Business, and One Hundred Years of Regulation* (New York: Knopf, 2003), chap. 2.

3   James G. Burrow, *AMA: Voice of American Medicine* (Baltimore: Johns Hopkins University Press, 1963); Hilts, *Protecting America's Health*, chaps. 1–3.

4   James Harvey Young, *The Medical Messiahs: A Social History of Medical Quackery in Twentieth-Century America* (Princeton, NJ: Princeton University Press, 1967).

5   Hilts, *Protecting America's Health*, 54–59.

6   Hilts, *Protecting America's Health*, 59.

7   Ibid.

8   U.S. Government Accountability Office, *Prescription Drugs: FDA's Oversight of the Promotion of Drugs for Off-Label Uses*, 2008.

9   Hilts, *Protecting America's Health*, 72–78.

10 Hilts, *Protecting America's Health*, 79–83.

11 Hilts, *Protecting America's Health*; Peter Temin, *Taking Your Medicine: Drug Regulation in the United States* (Cambridge, MA: Harvard University Press, 1980).

12 Temin, *Taking Your Medicine*.

13 Hilts, *Protecting America's Health*, 123.

14 In Hilts, *Protecting America's Health*, 125.

15 Hilts, *Protecting America's Health*, chaps. 6–8.

16 Hilts, *Protecting America's Health*, 127.

17 Hilts, *Protecting America's Health*, chap. 7; Henry A. Waxman, *The Marketing of Vioxx to Physicians*, memorandum to Democratic Members of the Government Reform Committee, May 5, 2005, http://oversight.house.gov/documents/20050505114932-41272.pdf.

18 Hilts, *Protecting America's Health*, 117.

19 Ibid., 115.

20 Richard Harris, *The Real Voice* (New York: Macmillan, 1964).

21 Melody Petersen, *Our Daily Meds* (New York: Farrar, Straus & Giroux, 2008), 123.

22 Hilts, *Protecting America's Health*, chap. 9; U.S. Office of the Inspector General, *FDA's Review Process for New Drug Applications: A Management Review*, March 2003.

23 Temin, *Taking Your Medicine*; Harry F. Dowling, *Medicines for Man: The Development, Regulation and Use of Prescription Drugs* (New York: Knopf, 1970), 86, chap. 8.

24 This account is based on Hilts, *Protecting America's Health*, chap. 10.

25 Hilts, *Protecting America's Health*, chap. 10.

26 Hilts, *Protecting America's Health*, 151.

27 This pattern of companies marketing drugs proven harmful in one country as harmless in others has been repeated over many years. See Milton Silverman, Philip R. Lee, and Mia Lydecker, *Prescriptions for Death: The Drugging of the Third World* (Berkeley: University of California Press, 1982); Milton Silverman, Mia Lydecker, and Philip R. Lee, *Bad Medicine: The Prescription Drug Industry in the Third World* (Stanford, CA: Stanford University Press, 1992); John Braithwaite, *Corporate Crime in the Pharmaceutical Industry* (London: Routledge & Kegan Paul, 1985); and BUKO, *Data and Facts 2004: German Drugs in the Third World* (Bielefeld, Germany: BUKO, 2004).

28 Hilts, *Protecting America's Health*, chap. 10.

29 Morton Mintz, "Heroine Of FDA Keeps Bad Drug Off Market," *Washington Post*, July 15, 1962.

30 Temin, *Taking Your Medicine*, 124–40.

31 Mintz, *By Prescription Only* (Boston: Beacon, 1967).

32 Hilts, *Protecting America's Health*, 168–73.

33 Ibid., chaps. 12–14.

34 Peter Lurie and Sidney M. Wolfe, *FDA Medical Officers Report Lower Standards Permit Dangerous Drug Approvals* (Washington, DC: Public Citizen, Health Research Group, 1998); U.S. Office of the Inspector General, *FDA's Review Process*, 2003; Public Citizen, "DO NOT USE! Lawsuit Reveals Serious Safety Problems with the Nonsteroidal Anti-inflammatory Drug Valdecoxib (BEXTRA)," *Worst Pills Best Pills Newsletter*, September 2004, 65–68.

35 William M. Wardell and Louis Lasagna, *Regulation and Drug Development* (Washington, DC: American Enterprise Institute, 1975); William M. Wardell, *Controlling the Use of Therapeutic Drugs: An International Comparison* (Washington, DC: American Enterprise Institute, 1978); Henry G. Grabowski, *Drug Regulation and Innovation: Empirical Evidence and Policy Options* (Washington, DC: American Enterprise Institute, 1976).

36 Industry-supported studies claimed that this presumptive lag in the regulatory review and approval of new drugs at the FDA in comparison to regulatory agencies in the United Kingdom, France, Spain, and Germany may have continued through 1999. See Kenneth I. Kaitin and Jeffrey S. Brown, "A Drug Lag Update," *Drug Information Journal* 29 (1995): 361–73.

37 Senate Select Committee on Small Business, *Competitive Problems in the Drug Industry: Drug Testing: Summary and Analysis* (Washington, DC: U.S. Government Printing Office, 1979).

38 Prescrire International, "A Look Back at Pharmaceuticals in 2006: Aggressive Advertising Cannot Hide the Absence of Therapeutic Advances," *Prescrire International* 16 (2007): 80–86.

39 Hilts, *Protecting America's Health*, 322.

40 U.S. General Accounting Office, *FDA Drug Approval: A Lengthy Process that Delays the Availability of Important New Drugs*, May 28, 1980, http://archive.gao.gov/d46t13/112450.pdf.

41 Jacob S. Hacker, *The Great Risk Shift: The Assault on American Jobs, Families, Health Care, and Retirement and How You Can Fight Back* (Oxford: Oxford University Press, 2006); Hilts, *Protecting America's Health*, chap. 14.

42 Hilts, *Protecting America's Health*, chap. 17.

43 Ibid., 315.

44 Ibid., 276–78.

45 Ibid., 296–98, chaps. 19–20.

46 Thomas J. Moore, *Prescription for Disaster: The Hidden Dangers in Your Medicine Cabinet* (New York: Simon & Schuster, 1998): 48–49.

47 Hilts, *Protecting America's Health*, 312.

48 Avery Johnson and Ron Winslow, "Drug Makers Say FDA Safety Focus Is Slowing New-Medicine Pipeline," *Wall Street Journal*, June 30, 2008.

49 Hilts, *Protecting America's Health*, 255–57.

50 Leslie Z. Benet, "Review and Critique of the Institute of Medicine Report, 'The Future of Drug Safety,'" *Clinical Pharmacology & Therapeutics* 81 (2007): 158–61.

51 Ibid.

52 Institute of Medicine, Committee on the Assessment of the US Drug Safety System, *The Future of Drug Safety: Promoting and Protecting the Health of the Public* (Washington, DC: National Academies Press, 2007), 194.

53 David Willman, "How a New Policy Led to Seven Deadly Drugs," *Los Angeles Times*, December 20, 2000.

54 Hilts, *Protecting America's Health*, chap. 21.

55 Institute of Medicine, *Future of Drug Safety*, 16.

56 Ibid., 23.

57 Institute of Medicine, *Future of Drug Safety*.

58 Ibid., 17.

59 Chris Adams and Alison Young, "Prescribing drugs 'off-label' is routine but can injure, kill patients"; "Drug-makers' promotions boost off-label use by doctors"; and "FDA oversight of 'off-label' drug use wanes as prescriptions rise," *McClatchy Newspaper*, November 2–4, 2003, http://www.mcclatchydc.com/244/story/28118.

html; 28119.html; and 29121.html.

60 Byron J. Richards, "How the FDA Is Becoming a Drug Company: Consumer Safety and Access to Natural Options Threatened," *Natural News.com*, June 14, 2007, http://naturalnews.com/021900.html.

61 Daniel Carpenter, Evan James Zucker, and Jerry Avorn, "Drug-Review Deadlines and Safety Problems," *New England Journal of Medicine* 358 (2008): 1354–61; Clark Nardinelli, Michael Lanthier, and Robert Temple, letter to the editor (response to "Drug-Review Deadlines"), *New England Journal of Medicine* 359 (2008): 95–98.

62 Laurence Landow, "FDA Approves Drugs Even When Experts on Its Advisory Panels Raise Safety Questions," *British Medical Journal* 318 (1999): 944; Michael A. Friedman et al., "The Safety of Newly Approved Medicines: Do Recent Market Removals Mean There Is a Problem?" *Journal of the American Medical Association* 281 (1999): 1728–34.

63 *Food and Drug Administration Amendments Act of 2007*, Public Law 110–85, 100th Cong. (September 27, 2007), *U.S. Statutes at Large* 121 (2007).

64 Bruce M. Psaty and David Korn, "Congress Responds to the IOM Drug Safety Report—In Full," *Journal of the American Medical Association* 298 (2008): 2185–87; Bruce M. Psaty and R. Alta Charo, "FDA Responds to Institute of Medicine Drug Safety Recommendations—In Part," *Journal of the American Medical Association* 297 (2007): 1917–19; Sheila Weiss Smith, "Sidelining Safety—the FDA's Inadequate Response to the IOM," *New England Journal of Medicine* 357 (2007): 960–63.

65 U.S. Food and Drug Administration, "Prescription Drug User Fee Act (PDUFA) IV: Drug Safety Five-Year Plan (Draft)," March 2008.

66 Institute of Medicine, *Future of Drug Safety*, 17.

67 Gardiner Harris, "The Safety Gap," *New York Times Magazine*, November 2, 2008.

68 Weiss Smith, "Sidelining Safety," 961.

69 Bridget M. Kuehn, "FDA's Science Infrastructure Failing," *Journal of the American Medical Association* 299 (2008): 157–58.

70 300 million people x 365 days x 4 cents a day = $4.38 billion. 2009 budget is $2.4 billion.

71 Mundy, "Grassley, Dingell Lead Calls."

72 Harris, "Safety Gap."

73 Code of Federal Regulations, *Title 21—Food and Drugs, Chapter I—Food and Drug Administration, Department of Health and Human Services, Subchapter D—Drugs for Human Use, Part 314—Applications for FDA Approval to Market a New Drug*, 21CFR314.50 (April 1, 2008).

74 Institute of Medicine, *Future of Drug Safety*, chap. 2.

75 Salomeh Keyhani, Marie Diener-West, and Neil Powe, "Are Development Times for Pharmaceuticals Increasing or Decreasing?" *Health Affairs* 25 (2006): 461–68.

76 For example, see the case in Merrill Goozner, *The $800 Million Pill: The Truth Behind the Cost of New Drugs* (Berkeley: University of California Press, 2004), chap. 1.

77 Donald W. Light, "Basic Research Funds to Discover Important New Drugs: Who Contributes How Much?" in *Monitoring Financial Flows for Health Research 2005: Behind the Global Numbers*, ed. Mary Anne Burke and Andrés de Francisco (Geneva: Global Forum for Health Research, 2006), 27–43.

78 Donald W. Light, "Misleading Congress about Drug Development," *Journal of Health Politics, Policy and Law* 32 (2007): 895–913.

79 Light, "Misleading Congress."

80 Salomeh Keyhani, Marie Diener-West, and Neil Powe, "Do Drug Prices Reflect Development Time and Government Investment?" *Medical Care* 43 (2005): 753–62.

81 Institute of Medicine, *Future of Drug Safety.*

82 Ibid., 59.

83 Arthur Atkinson et al., "Biomarkers and Surrogate Endpoints: Preferred Definitions and Conceptual Framework," *Clinical Pharmacological Therapy* 69 (2001): 89–95.

84 Food and Drug Administration, "Report on the Performance of Drugs and Biologics Firms in Conducting Postmarketing Commitment Studies," *Federal Register* 72, no. 22 (February 2, 2007): 5069–70, http://edocket.access.gpo.gov/2007/pdf/E7-1749.pdf

85 G. Singh and G. Triadafilopoulus, "Epidemiology of NSAID-induced GI Complications," *Journal of Rheumatology* 26, suppl. (1999): 18–24.

86 M. Michael Wolfe, David R. Lichtenstein, and Gurkirpal Singh, "Gastrointestinal Toxicity of Nonsteroidal Antiinflammatory Drugs," *New England Journal of Medicine* 340 (1999): 1888–99.

87 Weiss Smith, "Sidelining Safety," 960; Sheila Weiss Smith, author replies to letter to the editor (response to "Sidelining Safety"), *New England Journal of Medicine* 357 (2007): 2521–22.

CHAPTER THREE

The Commercialization
of Medical Decisions:
Physicians and Patients at Risk

HOWARD BRODY

Patients taking prescription drugs, as the chapters of this volume show, are at risk for adverse drug reactions, overtreatment, unsuitable treatment, disease mongering, and financial loss.

Who ought to protect patients from these risks? Chapter 2 shows how government (specifically the Food and Drug Administration [FDA] in the United States) is struggling to strengthen its weakened ability to protect the public and patients from private risks. If we are witnessing the privatization of risk, then we might next wonder if there are any *private* resources to which the patient/consumer might turn for protection.

The American medical profession has long viewed itself as just such a private resource, resolutely independent from either government or corporate dominance, dedicated to protecting public health and the interests of the patient. The special role of medicine is captured in the legal doctrine of the *learned intermediary*.[1] A person harmed by a prescription drug and another person harmed by an over-the-counter drug stand in different positions to the drugs' manufacturers under tort law. Other things equal, it will be harder for the patient to win a suit in the prescription-drug case because the physician writing the prescription should have used her extensive knowledge of medicine and pharmacology to protect the patient from possible harm. If harm occurs, the patient has an uphill battle proving that the manufacturer and not the physician should be liable.

American patients have been placed in an especially vulnerable position. At the same time as the corporate world and government have shifted risk onto the shoulders of individual citizens, their physicians—the main private resource that should be assisting them—have compromised their professionalism by having sales reps and favors bias their clinical judgment. The profession has, to a large extent, betrayed the public trust.[2] In other ways, the problem has arisen out of sight of the individual practitioner, as when medical journals publish articles that contain skewed or incomplete accounts of scientific studies, tilted to make the sponsor's drug look more effective or safer than it really is (as occurred extensively in the case of Vioxx described in Chapter 1).

To illuminate this compromised position of American physicians, this chapter explores the case of statin drugs used to lower cholesterol. Statins are viewed both as helpful drugs and as generally very safe. The fact that both physicians and patients think of statin drugs in this way, however, actually puts more patients at risk because tens of millions are prescribed statins for which there is no clear benefit to offset the risk of adverse reactions. The drugs' effectiveness in a relatively small group of patients has been extrapolated in an unscientific way to suggest equal effectiveness in a much larger population.

To illustrate how this can occur, I contrast two hypothetical physician-patient dialogues. One of these dialogues occurs commonly, while the other is rarely heard in today's medical practice. The dialogue based on scientific evidence that should take place between patients and their physicians differs markedly from the dialogue that usually does take place. The near absence of the evidence-based dialogue from everyday medical practice places millions of patients at risk in ways similar to those seen in the case studies elaborated in the other chapters. By not protecting patients from commercial misinformation and by acting on that misinformation, physicians put patients at greater risk than they would have been had they not turned to their physician for help. Fortunately, some recent events hint that medicine is beginning to reassert its own sense of professionalism, seeking once again to protect itself from commercial compromise and patients from the heightened risks of physician overtreatment so that trust in the profession can be restored.

TWO MEDICAL CHECKUPS

Imagine a middle-aged male patient seeing a physician for an annual checkup. He has no characteristics other than high cholesterol that put him at higher risk for heart attacks—he does not smoke, have high blood pressure or diabetes, or have relatives who have developed heart attacks at young ages. The patient, we imagine, tries to exercise and to eat a healthy diet, but with mixed results. Whether he could do better if he tried harder is unknown.

DIALOGUE A

DOCTOR A I'm pleased to say that I found nothing worrisome on physical examination, but your routine blood work that we had done last week shows a total cholesterol of 245, and your LDL or "bad" cholesterol is 140. If you look at this table from the Mayo Clinic health information Web site, you'll see that those values are considered "borderline high."

PATIENT A Darn, I really have been trying to exercise and eat right, just like you told me to.

DOCTOR A I think it's definitely time for a statin drug. These drugs have been proven to be very effective in lowering both total and LDL cholesterol. The vast majority of patients who take them experience no side effects. I've seen a few dedicated patients do really well at lowering their cholesterol with an aggressive diet and exercise program. But let's be realistic—few folks can stick with that sort of program for the long term.

PATIENT A Well, I guess you are right, though I really don't like the idea of taking a medicine every day when I'm not sick. Can I just take this for a while until my cholesterol goes down?

DOCTOR A No, I'd frankly expect this is basically going to be for life, unless you radically change your diet or exercise program. The minute you stop taking a statin your cholesterol goes right back up again.

PATIENT A My insurance requires a higher co-pay for brand-name drugs. Are any statins available as generics?

DOCTOR A Well, to tell you the truth, I was actually going to recommend a brand-name statin, Lipitor. My own experience with it has been very positive, and a few research studies show that it has certain advantages.

But, if truth be told, the important thing is that you get started on a statin for the high cholesterol that is putting you at risk. Exactly which statin is less important; and yes, there are a couple of generic statins available. I'll write you a script for generic lovastatin.[3]

PATIENT A Well, Doc, since the new medicine is going to do a good job of lowering my cholesterol, maybe I can treat myself to a cheeseburger and fries tonight, with chocolate cake for dessert? [*Laughs.*]

DOCTOR A Yes, it's tempting, isn't it? But you had better put that thought aside. After all, the whole idea here is for you to be healthier, right?

The average patient would probably have a high opinion of Doctor A following this visit. He showed he was interested in the patient's health. He did a thorough exam and ordered blood tests. He spent considerable time talking about the blood test results and options for treatment. He seems clearly motivated toward prevention. In the end, he prescribed the cheaper generic drug when asked. It might not bother the patient that Doctor A jumped quickly to drug treatment of cholesterol even though the blood tests came back borderline. At each step of the way, Doctor A gave reasons for recommending what he did, and each reason, taken by itself, sounded plausible.

Would Patient A's opinion change if he found out that Doctor A has extensive interactions with sales representatives from the pharmaceutical industry and relies on these representatives for a good deal of the information he possesses about drugs? And that, among the representatives that he sees, those from Pfizer (who makes Lipitor) form a considerable percentage?

If Doctor A did *not* have extensive interactions with the drug industry, he'd be quite unusual. A survey of U.S. physicians revealed that 94% reported some sort of relationship with the industry. Eighty-three percent accepted gifts from sales representatives ranging from pens, notepads, and coffee mugs to expensive dinners and trips to resort locations for conferences; 78% took promotional samples to give to patients; and 35% received reimbursements from industry as paid consultants or speakers.[4] With the new Code of Conduct in force, the gifts have become less prevalent.

Defenders of Doctor A might note that while he sees a lot of detail people from the firm that makes Lipitor, in the end he was happy to write a prescription for a different statin—one in fact that cost Patient A a lot less. Doesn't that show that he is not very much influenced by these sales tactics? One might even go so far as to suggest that it's good that Doctor A is quite eclectic in which detail people he sees and which gifts he takes. If he ends up seeing representatives from all the firms that make statins, any one firm's influence ought to be pretty much cancelled out.

Against this line of reasoning, consider who sent *no* detail people to try to "sell" Doctor A: sales reps for diet and exercise programs. It is not necessary to see detail people from only one among many drug firms to end up with a strong bias toward using drugs to treat problems that are just as amenable to non-drug therapy. But *is* a high cholesterol level amenable to treatment without drugs? Just what does the evidence say? Alternative voices are left out of the conversation.

DIALOGUE B

PATIENT B Since it's coming up on time for my annual checkup, I'd like you to go ahead and order my blood test for cholesterol, please.

DOCTOR B I would prefer not to.

PATIENT B Come again?

DOCTOR B I have read up on this issue and have done some thinking, and my conclusion now is that I should not routinely order cholesterol tests on patients.

PATIENT B But I thought that the official guidelines that you doctors are supposed to follow all recommend cholesterol testing.

DOCTOR B That's right, but I am now convinced that those guidelines are largely worthless because the people who write them are mostly paid consultants to the drug industry.[5] The scientific evidence does not support the guideline recommendations.

PATIENT B But if you don't know what my cholesterol level is, how can you tell me whether I need a statin drug?

DOCTOR B I can tell if you need a statin or not without any need to do a blood test because only certain categories of patients have been shown to benefit from statins. First, those who have already had a heart attack clearly do much better. That's the real high-payoff group. If you had had a heart attack, it would be my job to try to start you taking statins as soon afterward as you could swallow one.

The next group that seems to benefit from statins are people who have not yet had a heart attack but are at quite high risk for one — for instance, smokers with diabetes or with high blood pressure. But when we come to this group, it seems that the statin benefits, while not zero, are in fact miniscule. We characterize this in medical statistics by the "number needed to treat." We'd have to treat three hundred or four hundred of these high-risk men for several years in order to prevent one heart attack.[6] (The evidence for women benefitting from statins is much weaker.) So I try to explain this to men with those risk factors. And when I tell them, a good many choose not to start statins.

PATIENT B At least you do blood tests on those patients after you start them on statins, right? To be sure that you are reaching the targets for cholesterol lowering?

DOCTOR B No, I have stopped doing those tests too. The fact is that there has never been any compelling evidence that reaching any given target level with statin treatment leads to any better outcomes.[7]

PATIENT B But how, then, do you know how to adjust the doses of statins?

DOCTOR B I don't adjust the dose. The data that are available for the benefits of taking statins simply show that you accrue the benefit if you take the statin. The exact dose you take (or the target level of LDL that you reach) has not been shown to make any real difference in outcomes. I mean outcomes that matter to your health, like death or heart attack or stroke. We can always lower your numbers further by giving you a higher dose of statin. But that does not necessarily translate into less risk of heart disease.

PATIENT B This is all totally different from what I thought good medicine was. You are making my head spin.

DOCTOR B I know. I felt the same way at first. But the fact is that I think we have all been sold a bill of goods about managing cholesterol. Drug company marketing is not completely to blame for this, but it has been a big factor.

Dialogue B is based on a careful review of the cholesterol literature and independent analyses of the data in the original clinical trials of statins.[8] That so few physicians are even aware that this minority opinion exists attests to the extent to which the pharmaceutical industry and those who do its bidding have been able to monopolize medical information channels.

To summarize:

1. Statin drugs are very good at lowering one's blood-test numbers for both total and LDL cholesterol. But lowering numbers in the laboratory is not the goal of treatment. The real goal is to prevent serious events like a heart attack or stroke. Evidence experts call these "patient-oriented outcomes." Ignoring patient-oriented outcomes and focusing instead on improvements in laboratory numbers is one common technique employed by the industry to sell more drugs.

2. Statins are effective in reducing the risk of heart attack and stroke in patients with existing cardiovascular disease. In some high-risk patients with no known vessel disease, the statins are effective, but only with a very high "number needed to treat." Patient A does not fit into either of those categories.

3. Even where the therapeutic effect of statins is *present*, the size of the effect may be *low*. There is some evidence (admittedly not conclusive) that the beneficial effects of moderate exercise in preventing heart attacks may be several times greater than the effect of taking statins.[9]

4. There is very limited evidence, if any, that either the specific statin used or the dose affects benefits. The practice of using tests to monitor and make dosage adjustments once statins are started may therefore be a waste of time and money.

5. Recent research questions the scientific basis for much of today's widespread prescribing of statins and attests to the industry's ability to spin "facts" favorably. The results of the big JUPITER trial were used to advocate prescribing statins even to people with normal cholesterol levels; but the results actually indicated that cholesterol levels were irrelevant to identifying patients who could benefit from statins and that their benefits may be due to their anti-inflammatory

effects, not to their cholesterol-lowering properties at all.[10]

6. Brand-name statins are expensive and place the patient at significant financial risk, especially over a lifetime. The gradual shift to generic drugs reduces but does not eliminate the financial risk.

7. There are two major adverse effects of statins that affect a relatively small minority of those using them. The most serious but rare adverse effect is rhabdomyolysis, in which muscle fibers are broken down and the breakdown products are excreted in the urine. This is a medical emergency that in rare instances can be fatal. The less rare but still unusual adverse effect is a generalized weakness and achiness of the muscles. The problem with this second side effect is that it may not happen for months or years after the statin is started. This makes it hard for either the patient or the physician to associate it with taking a statin. Both adverse effects disappear once the statin is discontinued.

8. Besides causing symptoms, statins can cause silent damage to the liver. Guidelines generally recommend that to monitor patients for such damage (which fortunately also goes away once the statin is stopped), all patients receiving these drugs should have blood tests once or twice a year to check their liver status. Patients would still need these liver tests even if physicians no longer chose to do regular blood tests to check the cholesterol levels. So the cost of treatment (and the level of inconvenience for the patient) has to include these extra liver tests.

If Dialogue B is indeed an "evidence-based" account, why does one hardly ever hear it? First, the average patient might not trust a physician who said these things that are so much at odds with conventional wisdom. Everyone "knows" high cholesterol needs to be controlled, a piece of common sense that pharmaceutical companies did not create but have been quick to take advantage of. Pharmaceutical companies have spent a lot of advertising money to have everyone "know" this. Second, very few physicians are aware of this alternative view. The dominant story of the great benefits of using statins has been repeated to physicians by drug salespeople for two decades. The majority of medical journal articles about statins feature research sponsored by their manufacturers and are presented so as to stress the apparent benefits and downplay any doubts or limitations. Finally, as Doctor B noted, the official practice guidelines doctors are supposed to refer to—and that are increasingly used by insurance firms and other payers to determine whether physicians are paid a bonus for quality care—are often written by experts with financial ties to the drug industry.

TYPES OF PATIENT RISKS

The evidence shows that the decision to take statins is hardly as clear-cut as was presented by Doctor A. Patient A, we can now appreciate, was placed at risk in a number of ways. Even though the actual probability is low, he was placed at risk of *adverse drug reactions*, the potential dangerous side effects of drugs. Since the degree of benefit from statins in his case is likely to be very low, he was placed at risk for *unnecessary overtreatment* with a negative ratio of benefit to harm. He ran the risk of *inappropriate treatment* since diet and exercise counseling, which might well have been the most rational approach to managing his risks of coronary artery or blood-vessel disease, was displaced by a nearly exclusive focus on drug treatment. Finally, as we saw, Patient A was placed at risk for *financial loss* due to the high lifetime costs of statins (even generic ones).

What about *disease-mongering*, the promotion of drugs for conditions that pose no serious clinical threat? Patient A has become involved in a particular form of disease mongering that we might call *disease creep*. A few years ago, there was, by general agreement, one disease—coronary artery disease, of which a heart attack was an especially serious consequence. A person whose blood cholesterol level was high but who had no signs or symptoms of coronary artery disease had no detectable disease, even though he might be regarded as at future risk for developing a disease. But today, high cholesterol is considered a "disease." Ask people if they suffer from any diseases, and they may say, "I have high cholesterol." If Patient A looks in his medical chart, he will see in the medical "problem list" the entry "hypercholesterolemia." Further, the threshold for "high" cholesterol has been steadily lowered by a panel with industry ties. Each change adds millions who get a prescription they do not need and exposes them to adverse reactions.

The fact that the patient in the first dialogue now has a "disease" rather than simply a risk factor is, from Doctor A's point of view, financially advantageous. According to many insurance plans, if the physician puts down a code number for a disease in connection with an office visit, the insurance will pay the fee for the visit; if he does not, the patient pays cash. But the impact of the label "disease" is greater than just the question of coverage for the office visit. For example, in 2008, the American Academy of Pediatrics recommended that children as young as age 3 should be screened and those with high cholesterol should be medicated for life.[11] We have already seen how little evidence there is that middle-aged men at moderate risk for heart disease will derive any benefit from statin treatment, and this recommendation is even less based on good scientific evidence. The Academy's recommendation generated a storm of protest.[12] The recommendation illustrates the success of an industry-led campaign to define more life conditions as diseases and to define more and more people as "at risk" and in dire need of medications.[13] Chapters 4 and 5 provide additional examples of this trend. Because the FDA does little to prevent disease creep or the creation of new "diseases" or "risks" that pose little clinical danger, the risk and cost of undue promotions falls back on patients.

CAN DOCTORS SERVE AS PATIENT ADVOCATES?

With this privatization of risk from commercial promotions so thoroughly advanced, how might the medical profession fulfill the role of the "learned intermediary," advocating on behalf of the patient and compensating partially for the incredible power and wealth of the pharmaceutical industry? First, physicians and medical societies would avoid financial entanglements with pharmaceutical firms. Patients would then have confidence that the profession had not been bought off by the industry. Second, medicine would maintain a free flow of commercially unbiased information about the benefits and risks of pharmaceuticals, so that the individual practitioner had ready access to the best scientific evidence. As the historical case study of chloramphenicol and the more recent case of Vioxx illustrate, neither of these ideal conditions holds true.

Senator Charles Grassley (R-Iowa) spoke in Congress in July 2008 about his investigation of several prominent academic psychiatrists. Chapter 4 tells in detail the story of the industry-inspired over-prescription of psychotropic drugs. One of the areas in which the use of drugs among children has increased most rapidly is the use of major tranquilizers for bipolar disorder—a condition that was, a decade ago, seldom diagnosed in children. In order for the medical advice that patients and parents receive to be as trustworthy as possible, one would seek reassurance that this explosion in the prescribing of risky drugs for children was based solely on compelling scientific studies and not on any financial relationships with industry. It therefore undermined medicine's public trustworthiness when Senator Grassley revealed that two Harvard University psychiatrists who had been national leaders in calling for the expanded diagnosis of bipolar disorder in children and in treating it with antipsychotic (and incidentally, expensive brand-name) drugs had received generous payments from the manufacturers of the drugs, so generous ($1.6 million each) that they underreported to Harvard how much they received.[14]

We have already seen that 94% of U.S. physicians admit to accepting some gifts or payments from the pharmaceutical industry. The vast majority receive far lower sums than these few privileged academics (dubbed "key opinion leaders" by industry).[15] Nonetheless, it also seems clear that Senator Grassley did not have to dig very deep in order to discover newsworthy, egregious cases. A few months before Senator Grassley's revelations, a lawsuit against five manufacturers of implanted artificial joints was settled, revealing that some leading orthopedic surgeons had been paid a million dollars or more, ostensibly as consultants but more likely as a reward for frequent use of a manufacturer's product.[16] Multiple examples could be found indefinitely.

The U.S. pharmaceutical industry spends as much as $57 billion annually marketing drugs, with all but about $4 billion aimed directly at physicians.[17] Companies can readily purchase information on which physicians write how many prescriptions for each of their products (completely legal since no patient names are revealed). Armed with these prescribing data, sales representatives can dole out largesse in proportion to each physician's value to the company as a prescriber. Low prescribers may get only notepads and coffee mugs emblazoned with a drug logo. Higher prescribers will regularly be invited to dinners at luxury restaurants, perhaps even being paid as "consultants" merely to attend. Still higher prescribers will be hired as part of the company's speakers' bureau, supposedly because they have unique expertise in how to use the drug, but in actuality as yet one more financial reward for their prescribing practices.[18] An investigation in Minnesota, made possible by that state's sunshine law requiring the reporting of industry payments, revealed that fully one-quarter of the state's child psychiatrists are members of a company speakers' bureau, leaving us to wonder who might be left to constitute the audience.[19]

Social scientists can predict with confidence that these gifts will form a bond of reciprocity between the sales representative or company and the physician.[20] Normal human psychology creates an often subconscious impulse to give back to those who have given us gifts.[21]

FROM PRACTICE TO RESEARCH

We have seen many reasons to believe that the first essential condition for medicine protecting patients from the deleterious effects of risk privatization — independence from the financial embrace of the drug industry — has generally not been met. What about the second condition — maintaining a conduit for scientific evidence as free of commercial bias as possible?

Systematic reviews have concluded that commercial funding alone is a predictor of how "effective" a sponsor's drug appears to be, and approximately 80% of all clinical studies of drug treatment are funded by drug companies. On average, an industry-funded study is roughly four times more likely to conclude that the drug works and should be recommended than a study funded by a non-commercial organization.[22] A recent inquiry focused on studies in which one statin was compared to another statin. Such a study funded by one company was twenty times more likely to have results showing that that company's statin was superior to its competitor's yet thirty-five times more likely to recommend that statin over the competitor brand. The difference in these two numbers shows that nearly half the time, the *actual results contained in a research study fail to support the use of the drug.*[23] This suggests that even had Doctor A never spoken to a single drug rep, he might still have an unrealistic view of the superiority of one statin over another just from reading "scientific" articles in medical journals. Since the busy practitioner can find the recommendations to use the company's drug in the article's abstract but has to carefully read the entire paper to learn all the data, the study's sponsors can confidently predict that few physicians will ever note that the data don't support the recommendations.

The authors of this recent inquiry looked further into the designs of these statin-comparison studies and noted that the biased outcomes could be almost totally explained by certain design features of the studies. The most important design feature was inadequate blinding, or concealment, of which subject received which drug. This meant that the physicians assessing the outcomes often knew which drug each research subject was taking, a well-documented source of bias. If, for instance, a research subject developed vague, atypical chest pain, the physician could easily decide that this represented heart disease if she knew that the patient was taking the competitor statin. If she knew that this subject was assigned to the group taking the company's own statin, this same pain might be classified as a bad case of heartburn. In a study that involves thousands of subjects but has only a small percentage with bad outcomes, misclassifying just a handful of subjects can completely alter the results.

Other reviews of research studies have revealed numerous other means by which company-funded studies can be "cooked" or "spun" so as to increase the chances that the company's drug comes out looking good.[24] A very simple technique, for instance, is to compare one's own drug with an unrealistically low dose of a competitor's drug, to prove how well it works. By contrast, if the study is designed to show how many fewer side effects one's drug causes, one compares it to an unrealistically high dose of the competitor's drug.

The drug industry today regards the research that it funds as merely another form of marketing.[25] Journals read by pharmaceutical executives admonish them never to plan a single research study without their marketing team at the table alongside the scientists.[26] The scientists who allow the marketing agenda to overshadow any search for scientific truth may be the hired staff of the drug company, so that their loyalty is obvious. Alternatively, the scientists may be academic physicians appointed at major universities and medical centers. In the latter case, the willingness of the physicians to do industry's bidding, at the cost of obscuring the evidence base that their practitioner colleagues will rely on to prescribe rationally for their patients, is much less defensible.[27] Some academic physicians become tools of industry to assure continued company research funding, a more reliable source of research support today than increasingly scarce government and foundation grants. Others are seduced by the privileges of becoming a "key opinion leader" and being generously rewarded as a paid speaker and consultant.

If the scientists conducting the research too closely identify their interests with those of the sponsoring drug companies and minimize evidence of risks, where else can the public turn for protection? Medical journals, for example, ought to serve as citadels of good science, refusing to publish research papers that use biased samples, methods, and analysis. Sadly, the major journals have at least two big financial incentives to publish commercially sponsored research with little editorial oversight. First, pharmaceutical companies pay for the advertisements that keep most journals solvent and have been known to withdraw their advertising largesse from journals that seem opposed to company interests. More important, when a successful drug trial is published, the company typically purchases thousands of reprints of the article for distribution by its sales force. These reprints amount to almost pure profit for the journal.[28] Both the *New England Journal of Medicine* and the *Journal of the American Medical Association* allowed an underreporting of toxic side effects in major articles about the benefits of Vioxx and Celebrex, which then became key tools for massive prescribing of both. Merck paid the *New England Journal of Medicine* $900,000 for reprints of one article. It is very hard to detect exactly where the breakdowns occur in the editorial review process in such cases since journals treat their peer review systems as both confidential and proprietary and are very secretive about their inner workings. The end result, however, is that journals frequently fail to protect the medical consumer from the risks of drugs.

IS REFORM POSSIBLE?

The deleterious effects of the privatization of risk might have been mitigated if the medical profession had resolutely positioned itself on the side of public interest. Instead, medicine has gotten into bed with the pharmaceutical industry. In order to show how this has increased the risks faced by patients, I did not employ a case example such as Vioxx, which most everyone would agree represents a pharmaceutical failure, but instead looked at a case study that apparently represents a huge pharmaceutical and medical success — statin drugs for high cholesterol. I argued that the current way statins are commonly prescribed (Dialogue A) creates significant risks for patients. Dialogue B, which reduces those risks and is arguably more in line with scientific evidence, has been almost completely banished from the scene, thanks to aggressive industry marketing and control over the design and reporting of clinical trials.

As other chapters in this book demonstrate, the privatization of risk is a multifaceted problem that requires a number of solutions at different institutional levels. My focus in this chapter has been the specific role of the medical profession. What prospects for reform now exist that might better realign medicine with the interests of patients?

A few years ago, the medical profession seemed frozen in a state of denial and rationalization for its commercial ties. Even as evidence accumulated of the increasing influence of industry marketing over physician prescribing behavior and medical research outcomes, physicians continued to insist that they were thoughtful scientists who could not possibly be swayed by a few pens, coffee mugs, or slices of pizza.[29] Physicians' dependence on pharmaceutical sales representatives grew incrementally and imperceptibly throughout most of the twentieth century. Most physicians could not see this dependence as posing a problem for their profession.

Within a short span of time, however, the momentum appears to have changed direction. The major impetus for reform has emerged within academic medical centers. A number of leading academic physicians are calling for drastic changes in the environment of the medical center, including the near-banishment of sales reps with their gifts, food, and commercially biased messages.[30] A major motive for reform is the increased realization that *the physician's professionalism and integrity are at risk if action is not taken*. For decades, physicians have rationalized that they could have it both ways. They could continue to bask in the glow of public trust and respect that medicine had historically earned yet fill their pockets with the largesse of commercial enterprises that sought to influence their behavior in ways that would be viewed as an unacceptable conflict of interest if engaged in by judges or journalists.[31] Increasingly, medical leaders now realize that they must choose one path or the other and that maintaining trustworthiness in the eyes of the public will require avoiding most commercial entanglements.[32]

Action in Congress, made possible in part by the Democratic majority elected in 2006, has reinforced the call for greater professionalism and integrity within medicine in important ways. Senator Grassley and his colleagues, by investigating prominent academic physicians and their financial conflicts of interest, send two messages to the profession. First, they remind academic medical leaders that there will be serious consequences, in the form of public embarrassment, to maintaining the status quo. Second, they inform medicine of a shift in public opinion and an increased level of public scrutiny. Senator Grassley, we must assume, would not be targeting these high-rolling academic physicians unless this scored points with the voting public. And indeed, polls indicate that the public is concerned about medical conflict of interest and would favor legislation to limit and expose industry payments to physicians.[33] This in turn reinforces professional fears that public trust will be jeopardized unless reforms are implemented.

Academic leaders, on the other hand, are not representative of rank and file medical practitioners. In June 2008, the Council on Ethical and Judicial Affairs of the American Medical Association (AMA) recommended a significant modification in the AMA code of ethics to prohibit many forms of gifts from the pharmaceutical industry. The response of the AMA House of Delegates was to refer the measure back to committee — an indication that the zeal for reform was not shared by many who represent the average practitioner.[34] The National Physicians Alliance has launched an Unbranded Doctor campaign to provide materials and resources especially for the private physicians' office that wishes to divest itself of the influence and the presence of pharmaceutical marketing, drug samples, and so on.[35]

How is the pharmaceutical industry responding to these challenges to its customary business model? A few defenders of the industry within academic centers have decried the new policies, claiming that the commercialization of academic medicine is essential to spur innovation and condemning ethical concerns over conflicts of interest as silly exercises in political correctness.[36] The industry's response, released by the Pharmaceutical Research and Manufacturers of America (PhRMA) in July 2008, was a newly revised Code on Interactions with Healthcare Professionals, replacing a generally ineffectual code of ethics from 2002.[37] At one level, the new Code appears to be a principled response to critics of industry marketing aimed at physicians. The Code insists that the ultimate objective should be the exchange of educational and scientific information between the industry and the medical profession. The Code restricts or bans activities that do not further that objective—even going so far as to propose the elimination of the now ubiquitous "reminder items" such as pens, coffee mugs, and notepads covered with drug logos. PhRMA plans to create a Web site on which the names of companies that agree to adhere to the Code will be posted and promises to outline a method for the external audit of compliance.

PhRMA critics, however, immediately noted that this Code, like all previous ones, is completely voluntary and leaves intact most of the essential methods by which the industry now influences physician prescribing. Sponsored lectures over meals, sales rep visits to physicians, industry-sponsored continuing medical education, and companies' purchase of physician prescribing data would all continue.[38] The new Code looks more like window dressing in front of the ongoing commercialization of professional judgment.

What is most likely the true intent of the new Code (if past industry behavior is any guide) was revealed in the Massachusetts House of Representatives a week later.[39] The state Senate had passed a bill to rein in health care costs that included several restrictions on pharmaceutical marketing—a ban on gifts and meals to physicians, a ban on physician prescribing data, and a sunshine requirement that all company payments to physicians be publicly reported. The version that passed the House eliminated the gift ban and sunshine clause and delayed the ban on prescribing data by a year. The House, it was reported, responded to drug industry lobbyists' claims that the new Code would effectively eliminate the excesses of industry marketing on a voluntary basis, so that restrictive state legislation was not needed.

At the federal level, Senator Grassley's investigations of physicians' conflicts of interest are tied to the bill before his committee, the Physician Payments Sunshine Act, which would require federal reporting by drug and medical device makers of gifts and payments to physicians.[40] PhRMA indicated its support of this legislation, apparently in hopes of heading off further sunshine efforts at the state level. However, pharmaceutical lobbying has already weakened a number of provisions of the federal legislation.[41] The industry has positioned itself to exert its will on the new Democratic-controlled Congress; campaign contributions previously directed almost exclusively to Republicans are now being redistributed to the majority party.[42]

The industry's combined public relations and lobbying strategy has been successful in the past. The public face that the industry presents is that of promoting the highest ethical and scientific standards in its quest to discover new lifesaving drugs. Behind the scenes, and aided by this benign public image, one of Washington's largest contingents of lobbyists works hard to delay or to emasculate any legislation that might force the industry to change its profitable marketing methods. Legislation the industry opposes is seldom openly defeated after a loud floor debate in Congress; instead it simply disappears into a committee room and never emerges.

CONCLUSION

Through its traditional professional oath of fidelity to the interests of the patient, medicine has promised to remain financially and scientifically independent of commercial entities like the pharmaceutical industry. To date, this promise has not been kept. Keeping the promise in the future requires the medical profession to step up as a key player but cannot rely on the profession alone. Both professional and legal-regulatory reforms will be required if the public is to be adequately protected from all the risks we have identified.

NOTES

1   Gerald S. Schatz and Howard Brody, "Letter: Learned Intermediary Doctrine," *Federal Lawyer* 53 (2006): 8–9.

2   Howard Brody, *Hooked: Ethics, the Medical Profession, and the Pharmaceutical Industry* (Lanham, MD: Rowman and Littlefield, 2007); Jerome P. Kassirer, *On the Take: How Medicine's Complicity with Big Business Can Endanger Your Health* (New York: Oxford University Press, 2005).

3   If the patient did a little price-checking at a popular pharmacy Web site, he would find that 100 tablets of a commonly used dose of Lipitor cost $357.00 while the equivalent lovastatin prescription costs $66.64.

4   Eric G. Campbell et al., "A National Survey of Physician-Industry Relationships,"

New England Journal of Medicine 356, no. 17 (2007): 1742–50.

5   Niteesh K. Choudhry, Henry Thomas Stelfox, and Allan S. Detsky, "Relationships Between Authors of Clinical Practice Guidelines and the Pharmaceutical Industry," *Journal of the American Medical Association* 287, no. 5 (2002): 612–17.

6   John Carey, "Do Cholesterol Drugs Do Any Good?" *Business Week*, January 28, 2008, 52.

7   Therapeutics Initiative, "Statin's Benefit for Secondary Prevention Confirmed. What Is the Optimal Dosing Strategy?" *Therapeutics Letter* (University of British Columbia) 49 (July–September 2003), http://www.ti.ubc.ca/node/51 (accessed July 19, 2008).

8   J. Abramson and J.M. Wright, "Are Lipid-Lowering Guidelines Evidence-Based?" *Lancet* 369 (2007): 168–69.

9   John Abramson, *Overdosed America* (New York: HarperCollins, 2004).

10 P.M. Ridker et al., "Rosuvastatin to Prevent Vascular Events in Men and Women with Elevated C-Reactive Protein," *New England Journal of Medicine* 359 (2008): 2195–2207: O. Melander et al, "Novel and Conventional Biomarkers for Prediction of Incident Cardiovascular Events in the Community," *Journal of the American Medical Association* 302 (2009): 49–57.

11 Tara Parker-Pope, "Cholesterol Screening Is Urged for Young," *New York Times*, July 7, 2008.

12 Alan Zarembo, "Use of Statins in Children Debated," *Los Angeles Times*, July 9, 2008.

13 Ray Moynihan and Alan Cassels, *Selling Sickness: How the World's Biggest Pharmaceutical Companies Are Turning Us All into Patients* (New York: Nation Books, 2005).

14 Benedict Carey and Gardiner Harris, "Psychiatric Association Faces Senate Scrutiny Over Drug Industry Ties," *New York Times*, July 12, 2008.

15 Ray Moynihan, "Key Opinion Leaders: Independent Experts Or Drug Representatives in Disguise?" *British Medical Journal* 336 (2008): 1402–3.

16 Barnaby J. Feder, "New Focus of Inquiry Into Bribes: Doctors," *New York Times*, March 22, 2008.

17 Marc-André Gagnon and Joel Lexchin, "The Cost of Pushing Pills: A New Estimate of Pharmaceutical Promotion Expenditures in the United States," *PLoS Medicine* 5, no. 1: e1.

18 Daniel Carlat, "Dr. Drug Rep," *New York Times Magazine*, November 25, 2007.

19 Gardiner Harris, Benedict Carey, and Janet Roberts, "Psychiatrists, Children and Drug Industry's Role," *New York Times*, May 10, 2007.

20 Jason Dana and George Loewenstein, "A Social Science Perspective on Gifts to

Physicians from Industry," *Journal of the American Medical Association* 290 (2003): 252–55.

21 M. D. Rawlins, "Doctors and the Drug Makers," *Lancet* 2, no. 8406 (1984): 814; Marcia Angell, *The Truth About the Drug Companies: How They Deceive Us and What to Do About It* (New York: Random House, 2004).

22 Joel Lexchin et al., "Pharmaceutical Industry Sponsorship and Research Outcome and Quality: Systematic Review," *British Medical Journal* 326 (2003): 1167–70.

23 Lisa Bero et. al., "Factors Associated with Findings of Published Trials of Drug-Drug Comparisons: Why Some Statins Appear More Efficacious than Others," *PLoS Medicine* 4, no. 6 (2007): e184.

24 Daniel J. Safer, "Design and Reporting Modifications in Industry-Sponsored Comparative Psychopharmacology Trials," *Journal of Nervous and Mental Disease* 190 (2002): 583–92.

25 Melody Petersen, "Madison Ave. Plays Growing Role in Drug Research," *New York Times*, November 22, 2002.

26 Elisabeth Pena, "Building Bridges: Bringing R&D and Marketing Closer," *Pharma-VOICE*, 2004 (May): 8–13.

27 Sheldon Krimsky, *Science in the Private Interest: Has the Lure of Profits Corrupted Biomedical Research?* (Lanham, MD: Rowman and Littlefield, 2003).

28 Richard Smith, "Medical Journals Are an Extension of the Marketing Arm of Pharmaceutical Companies," *PLoS Medicine* 2, no. 5 (2005): e138.

29 Bert Spilker, "The Benefits and Risks of a Pack of M&Ms: A Pharmaceutical Spokesman Answers His Industry's Critics," *Health Affairs* 21, no. 2 (2002): 243–44; Susan Chimonas, Troyen Brennan, and David Rothman, "Physicians and Drug Representatives: Exploring the Dynamics of the Relationship," *Journal of General Internal Medicine* 22 (2007): 184–90.

30 Troyen Brennan et al., "Health Industry Practices That Create Conflicts of Interest: A Policy Proposal for Academic Medical Centers," *Journal of the American Medical Association* 295 (2006): 429–33.

31 Jerome P. Kassirer, *On the Take: How Medicine's Complicity with Big Business Can Endanger Your Health* (New York: Oxford University Press, 2005).

32 Association of American Medical Colleges, *Report of the AAMC Task Force on Industry Funding of Medical Education to the AAMC Executive Council*, April 27, 2008, http://www.aamc.org/research/coi/industryfunding.pdf (accessed June 8, 2008).

33 International Communications Research, *The Prescription Project* (Media, PA: June 2008), http://www.prescriptionproject.org/assets/pdfs/Prescripton%20Project%20Survey_0618.pdf (accessed July 18, 2008).

34   Andis Robeznieks, "Getting Down to Business: AMA Members Look at Group's Own Relevance," *Modern Healthcare* 2008 (June 23): 10.

35   National Physicians Alliance, "The Unbranded Doctor Campaign," http://npalliance.org/pages/the_unbranded_doctor_campaign (accessed July 18, 2008).

36   Thomas P. Stossel, "Regulating Academic-Industrial Research Relationships—Solving Problems or Stifling Progress?" *New England Journal of Medicine* 353 (2005): 1060–65; Richard Allen Epstein, "Conflicts of Interest in Health Care: Who Guards the Guardians?" *Perspectives in Biology and Medicine* 50 (2007): 72–88.

37   Pharmaceutical Research and Manufacturers of America, *Code on Interactions with Healthcare Professionals*, July 2008, http://www.phrma.org/files/PhRMA%20Marketing%20Code%202008.pdf (accessed July 19, 2008).

38   Gardiner Harris, "Drug Industry to Announce Revised Code on Marketing," *New York Times*, July 10, 2008.

39   Kay Lazar, "Panel Rejects Ban on Drug Firm Gifts; Deletes Bill's Disclosure Requirements," *Boston Globe*, July 16, 2008.

40   Pew Prescription Project, "The Physicians Payment Sunshine Act (S.301) and Vermont's 2009 Gifts Ban and Disclosure Law (S.48)," *Fact Sheet* (Boston: Prescription Project, June 16, 2009), http://www.prescriptionproject.org/tools/sunshine_docs/files/0013.pdf (accessed July 3 2009).

41   Howard Brody, "Federal Sunshine Bills—Where Do We Stand," Hooked: Ethics, Medicine, and Pharma blog, May 31, 2008, http://brodyhooked.blogspot.com/2008/05/federal-sunshine-bills-where-do-we.html (accessed July 23, 2008).

42   Jeffrey H. Birnbaum, "Drug Firms Woo Democrats, Helping Defeat Their Bills," *Washington Post*, March 12, 2008.

CHAPTER FOUR

Pharmaceuticals and the Medicalization of Social Life

ALLAN V. HORWITZ

An enormous change has occurred over the past twenty years in how Americans perceive and treat psychological and behavioral problems. In particular, the 1990s and the first decade of the twenty-first century have seen a dramatic upsurge in the medicalization of social life. Medicalization means that some condition is defined as a medical problem and is treated through medical techniques.[1] Troubles that had been viewed as spiritual, moral, or behavioral problems and handled through prayer, counseling, or punishment or simply tolerated are now defined as diseases and addressed through biomedical treatments that physicians provide. Especially since 1997, when pharmaceutical companies were permitted to advertise their products directly to consumers, medicalization has become almost completely associated with the use of chemicals that alter presumably defective biological conditions.

Drugs offer the promise of fast, easy, and effective control of many kinds of distress and deviant behavior. They can sometimes enhance personal functioning, prevent minor problems from becoming more serious, and be more cost effective than alternatives. Yet, drug use also entails many drawbacks. No drug is perfectly safe, and all drugs create side effects for a proportion of their users. These effects can sometimes be very severe and are occasionally life-threatening. When used for long periods of time, drugs carry the risk of dependency. Employing drugs as first-line treatments can also forestall consideration of other, possibly more effective treatment strategies. It can also deflect attention away from the role of social conditions, on the one hand, or individual responsibility, on the other, in the creation of personal problems.

This chapter considers some recent developments surrounding medicalization, in particular, the dramatic upsurge in the use of pharmaceuticals to treat a variety of psychosocial problems. Because different kinds of problems are usually related to the period of life when they develop—childhood and adolescence, adulthood, and old age—we consider each life stage separately. While medicalization has undoubtedly brought benefits to many, it also has created dangers that too often are hidden and unacknowledged. Governmental bodies such as the Food and Drug Administration (FDA) have only exerted control over the pharmaceutical industry on rare occasions in recent years, so that consumers themselves have borne the risks that regimes of medication entail.

MEDICATING CHILDREN AND ADOLESCENTS

The most dramatic recent changes in medicalization have occurred among children and adolescents. The past decade, in particular, has seen an explosive growth in the use of pharmaceuticals to control behavioral and emotional problems among the young. Especially serious risks accompany the increasing medicalization of childhood troubles.

Attention Deficit Hyperactivity Disorder (ADHD) has become a highly prevalent psychiatric condition among children and adolescents. Just twenty years ago, less than 1% of children were diagnosed and treated with ADHD.[2] By 2003, however, 7.8% of youth aged 4 to 17 years received an ADHD diagnosis, and 4.3% took medication for this disorder.[3] Most treatment for ADHD involves the use of stimulant drugs, in particular, amphetamines. Over two million children now receive these drugs each year.[4] Their rising use is especially apparent in the government-funded Medicaid program, where spending for stimulants grew almost ninefold in inflation-adjusted dollars between 1991 and 2001.[5] The use of drugs to control children's behavior and emotions, although growing worldwide, is mainly an American phenomenon: the United States uses over 80% of the world's supply of stimulants.[6]

The pervasive use of stimulant drugs among children poses several risks. Widespread concern exists that many medicated children do not, in fact, have a psychiatric condition but instead behave badly, irritate teachers, and frustrate parents. The criteria for ADHD found in the official manual of the psychiatric profession, the *Diagnostic and Statistical Manual of Mental Disorders* (DSM),[7] are very general and have considerable overlap with natural processes of inattention, distraction, and boisterousness. One leading expert on ADHD estimates that only about 10% of current youthful users would require medication if they had optimal family and school situations.[8] Findings that the majority of children receiving stimulants are not functionally impaired suggest that such concerns are well-founded.[9]

Although stimulant drugs are safe for most users, some suffer side effects that can include decreased appetite, sleep difficulties, depression, headaches, and stomach upset. At the extreme, a number of children suffer psychotic reactions or toxic overdoses from the use of these drugs. It is also troubling that the long-term impacts from chronic stimulant use are unknown. Another source of unease is that as rates of drug use rise, treatments that do not involve medication decline.[10] The medicalization of childhood behavior problems tends to shut off alternative behavioral, psychosocial, and educational responses.

American children are being diagnosed with and treated for not only mounting numbers of behavior problems but also depression, at alarmingly growing rates. Government figures show that about one in ten teenagers, or 2.2 million, had a Major Depressive Disorder (MDD) in 2004.[11] The period from 1994 to 2001 witnessed a stunning 250% increase in the number of visits to physicians that resulted in a prescription for psychotropic medication among adolescents.[12] Antidepressant use in this group has grown even faster, swelling from three- to fivefold since the early 1990s, with especially accelerated rates after 1999.[13]

This precipitous rise in antidepressant use should set off a number of alarms. First, like the ADHD diagnoses, the DSM criteria for MDD do not distinguish intense but normal sadness that can arise from breaking up with a boyfriend or girlfriend, failing an important test, or getting punished by parents from depressive disorders. Many young people who are responding to stressful circumstances might be mistakenly labeled as depressed and unnecessarily medicated. Even when MDD diagnoses are appropriate, antidepressants might not be an effective tool for treating depression among children and adolescents. One large analysis of all studies of this question among preteens indicates that improvement among those who are medicated barely exceeds placebo treatment: 58% of children respond to placebo compared to 65% who receive active medication.[14] All antidepressants have adverse reactions, and these can be especially potent among the young. Because the widespread use of antidepressants among the young is so new, no studies are available about risks of adverse effects from their long-term use.

A particular concern lies in possible increased risk of suicidal behavior among young people who take antidepressants. Several studies show reports of suicidal ideation and/or behavior are greater among those taking antidepressants than those who receive placebos.[15] One important case control study of children and adolescents aged 6 to 18 who were hospitalized for depression showed that youths treated with antidepressants had 1.52 times more suicide attempts or deaths from suicide than those who did not receive antidepressant drugs.[16]

Concern over heightened risk of child and adolescent suicidal potential from antidepressant use led the FDA to undertake an exhaustive review of the issue. Although the FDA review found that none of the 2,200 children taking antidepressants who were covered in the review actually completed suicide, they were about twice as likely as those in placebo groups to experience suicidal thinking or to make suicide attempts.[17] In response, in 2006 the FDA uncommonly stood up to the pharmaceutical industry and adopted a "black box warning label," the most serious type of warning in prescription drug labeling, indicating that antidepressants may increase the risk of suicidal thinking and behavior in some children and adolescents. These concerns have also led regulatory agencies in Great Britain to warn physicians not to prescribe most antidepressant medications to anyone younger than 18.

Another disquieting possibility is that published reports minimize the number of adverse reactions associated with antidepressant use among the young. In 2004, the then-attorney general of New York State, Eliot Spitzer, filed a lawsuit charging the drug firm GlaxoSmithKline (GSK) with fraud for failing to report that adolescents who took Paxil had higher rates of suicidal ideation than those on placebo.[18] In addition, the suit alleged that the company failed to publish data that indicated Paxil was no more effective than placebo in treating depression. Published studies, therefore, might underestimate the cost/benefit ratio of antidepressant (and other drug) use.

Despite the dangers involved in the steep increase in stimulants and antidepressants, the most worrisome trend in the medicalization of child and adolescent problems is the alarming increase in the use of the strongest psychotropic drugs — the antipsychotics. The number of persons 20 years old and younger who received a prescription for an antipsychotic medication jumped from about 200,000 in 1993–95 to about 1,225,000 in 2002, a more than sixfold increase in less than a decade.[19] This trend is particularly worrisome because there is no evidence that these drugs can be used safely with this age group. Instead, physicians are adopting practices established for adults and applying them without justification to children and adolescents. The few studies that exist suggest that negative side effects, including weight gain, diabetes, and involuntary movement disorders, might be worse for children and adolescents than for adults.[20] Nevertheless, the use of antipsychotic drugs among youth continues to grow despite the absence of evidence for either their safety or their effectiveness.

The spectacular rise in rates of bipolar (or manic-depressive) disorder in youth provides the most dramatic instance of the "discovery" of a new childhood mental disorder. This disorder was traditionally thought to arise in midlife and until recently was virtually unknown among youth. Then, in 2007 a national survey discovered an astonishing *fortyfold* increase in the number of children and adolescents treated for bipolar disorder from 1994 to 2003.[21] The criteria for pediatric bipolar disorder are so vague and the diagnosis is subject to so many uncertainties that many experts even question the existence of the disorder at all.[22] The common denominator among children treated for this condition seems to be that their conduct is extremely disturbing to adults, usually their parents and/or teachers. Pediatric bipolar diagnoses and resulting prescriptions for medication are often used as a way of pacifying disruptive behavior. Given the lack of data for treatment efficacy, the strong adverse side effects from powerful medications, and the great potential for abuse this diagnosis poses, the risks from this diagnosis seem to far exceed its possible benefits.

It is unlikely to be coincidental that the vast increase in diagnoses and prescriptions among the young has occurred at the same time as older psychotropic medications were coming off their patents. The income from once hugely profitable drugs plunges after their patents expire and generics enter the market.[23] This forces drug companies to adapt old medications to new, patentable uses or to find new populations, such as ever-younger users, for their products. Skepticism over the legitimacy of the pediatric bipolar diagnosis and resulting medication treatments is fueled by the fact that their leading promoter, child psychiatrist Joseph Biederman, has received at least $1.6 million in consulting fees from the drug industry in recent years.[24] The result, in all likelihood, is that millions of young people are at risk for careers of drug use for disorders that barely existed ten years ago.

Normal but distressing and disruptive childhood behaviors are increasingly being labeled as mental disorders. Children have always behaved in ways that annoy and frustrate their parents, disturb their teachers, and are distressing to themselves. Only very recently, however, have these behaviors been considered to be mental disorders that must be treated with medications. Moreover, the emphasis on medication forecloses alternative ways of handling behavioral and learning problems that not only pose fewer risks but also can be more effective than medication. While many hyperactive and depressed children have disorders and benefit from drug treatments, others who are labeled and treated do not have mental disorders at all.

SCREENING FOR CHILDHOOD AND ADOLESCENT MENTAL HEALTH PROBLEMS

The huge and growing rate of drug treatments could be only the tip of the medicalizing iceberg among the young. Many mental health professionals believe that child and adolescent disorders are seriously underrecognized and undertreated. They have launched large-scale efforts that attempt to screen, in principle, every child and adolescent in the United States for signs of mental illness. In 2003 the President's New Freedom Commission Report recommended that "every child should be screened for mental illness once in their youth in order to identify mental illness and prevent suicide among youth."[25] A number of state legislatures have adopted measures that aim to implement this goal.

The impetus for screening lies in the findings that most young people that psychiatrists might regard as having a mental illness don't get treatment for it. The lack of treatment, in turn, is seen as perpetuating suffering and behavioral problems and limiting educational achievement. As well, untreated minor conditions are assumed to develop into more serious, recurring, and chronic diseases. In the worst case scenario, untreated mental illnesses can lead to horrific outcomes such as suicide or school shootings. Advocates of screening argue that, because the first symptoms of depression often develop among children and adolescents, the most effective prevention would take place as early as possible.

To deal with the enormous perceived amount of unidentified mental illness, the screening movement has developed short screening scales for administration in school classrooms that ask students whether they have experienced a variety of distressing symptoms of sadness, anxiety, problems from substance abuse, and the like. Students who report enough of these symptoms are then referred to a mental health professional for a more extensive psychiatric interview and, if necessary, a referral into psychiatric treatment. Pharmaceutical companies have sponsored the development of many screening measures, which promise to open previously untapped markets of potential drug users.

Screening scales ask questions such as "In the past six months, were there times when you were very sad?" or "In the past six months, has there been a time when you weren't interested in anything and felt bored or just sat around most of the time?" Positive answers to enough of these common feelings are supposed to lead to an interview with a mental health professional. The symptoms screening scales contain are common enough so that about a quarter of all students screened, which rises to nearly half in some schools, are considered to have problems that warrant a follow-up interview.

The broad nature of the questions on these scales ensures that many adolescents who are experiencing normal emotions will mistakenly be considered to suffer from a mental disorder. Indeed, the number of youths who score positively for potential mental illness on the screening instrument but are not considered to have a mental illness in a follow-up interview exceeds 80%. In addition, the kinds of symptoms these scales assess are highly sensitive to such transitory yet commonly occurring phenomena as the breakup of a romantic relationship, arguing with parents, or losing a crucial game in sports. Their ephemeral nature is illustrated by the fact that when asked the same questions about symptoms at eight-day intervals, only about half the students who provide positive answers the first time give the same answer only a week later.

There are many dangers of treating distressing but normal and transitory emotions as signs of mental illness. One is that an enormous number of young people will be identified as having the potential to develop a major mental disorder and be at risk for suicidal behaviors. Most of these labels, at least four of every five, will be false. Yet, such labels suggest a rethinking of the nature of the identified adolescents not just to themselves but also to their parents, their teachers, and their peers. The resulting amount of stigma is unknown but is likely to be substantial in many cases.

Identifying an adolescent with mental illness is supposed to result in a referral for professional treatment. Given current trends, such referrals are likely to involve medications. As noted above, many unanswered questions exist about whether antidepressant medication works effectively in teenagers, and most studies do not show that their benefits exceed those of placebo. Likewise, drugs pose greater risks for children and adolescents than adults, including heightened suicidal ideation and the unknown impact of instituting long-term medication regimens at early ages.

One of the major goals of the screening movement is to identify students who are at high risk for particularly dire outcomes such as suicide or school shootings. Yet, there is no evidence that screening successfully targets the tiny number of individuals who become actively suicidal or homicidal. In a number of school shootings, the perpetrators were already using antidepressant drugs, which at least some experts believe might have contributed to their murderous states of mind.[26] Other experts believe that antidepressant medications raise, rather than lower, the probability of suicide among adolescents.[27] The questionable effectiveness of antidepressants for young people coupled with their adverse effects indicates that skepticism toward sweeping screening programs is appropriate until far more information is available about their benefits and risks.

Moreover, advocates of screening programs do not seriously consider the burdens on the mental health system of adopting the kind of

; program that would administer a screening scale to "every" ıt in the United States. Literally millions of young people would nental health system that is in no way equipped to handle and treat such massive numbers of cases, many of whom do not in all likelihood have a mental disorder at all. The probable result would be a massive increase in the administration of psychotropic drugs, with possibly dire future mental health consequences.

Perhaps the major failure of the screening movement lies in its assumption that any distressing feelings are abnormal and must be monitored, classified, and controlled to prevent even transient distress and role impairment. Remarkably, not a single study demonstrates that screening programs actually improve mental health outcomes or prevent suicide. No evidence currently exists that their possible benefits override the risks of inappropriate diagnosis, unnecessary and possibly harmful treatment, and stigma.

THE MEDICALIZATION OF ADULT PSYCHOSOCIAL PROBLEMS

The latest figures on rates of presumed mental disorders among adults are striking.[28] They show that at some point in their lives a fifth of Americans have had mood disorders, a quarter impulse control disorders, and nearly a third anxiety disorders. Overall, about half of adults have had some mental illness. These figures are considerably higher than rates found in surveys taken before the 1990s. It is doubtful that the mounting numbers of people considered to be mentally ill stem from an actual increase in these conditions. Instead, they are more likely to reflect the use of measures that treat natural but highly distressing emotions as well as mental disorders as signs of illness.

The pharmaceutical industry has exploited the large numbers of presumably mentally ill people, using their advertising, marketing, and educational campaigns. Correspondingly, there has been a sharp increase in the number of prescriptions written for psychotropic drugs. During the last decade of the twentieth century, the psychiatric drug market grew by a phenomenal 638% in the United States.[29] The development and intensive marketing of selective serotonin reuptake inhibitors (SSRIs) in the late 1980s were largely responsible for this growth. By the turn of the century, spending on psychotropic drugs had reached $20 billion annually. At this time, three of the top seven bestselling drugs of any sort (Prozac, Paxil, Zoloft) were antidepressants. Three examples illustrate the explosive growth in medicalization among adults: major depressive disorder, social anxiety disorder, and sexual dysfunctional disorder.

MAJOR DEPRESSIVE DISORDER

Major Depressive Disorder (MDD) is the most common diagnosis among adults in psychiatric treatment. Its symptoms include states of low mood, diminished pleasure, sleep and appetite difficulties, fatigue, and lack of concentration. Studies estimate that about 17% of persons suffer from MDD over their lifetime, and about 7% during a one-year period.[30] Do all these people have a serious mental disorder, or are they suffering from normal, but intense, emotions of sadness?

The major problem in evaluating rates of MDD is that the same symptoms of feeling down, low energy, difficulties with sleeping and eating, and the like also can indicate normal responses to some serious loss.[31] For example, the diagnostic criteria for MDD exempt cases of grief after the death of a loved one that are not prolonged even if they otherwise meet the criteria. This is because intense bereavement after an intimate dies is a normal human emotion, not a mental disorder. Yet, the criteria do not exempt comparable situations that involve, for example, intense episodes of sadness that last two weeks or more after the breakup of a marriage, the unexpected loss of a valued job, or the discovery that an intimate has a life-threatening illness. In other cases, reported symptoms could be normal responses to long-standing conditions of poverty, chronic marital problems, or injustice. But the DSM diagnostic criteria consider persons who report enough "symptoms" after losses other than bereavement as mentally ill and in need of mental health treatment even if their low moods are responses to losses and hardship and go away when these stressors abate.

Defining normal sadness as depressive mental disorder has contributed to the medicalization of distress that expectably results from social circumstances. Because most people who report enough symptoms to be considered as having a depressive disorder do not seek mental health treatment, they are considered to have an "unmet" need for treatment. Mental health policy, media reports, and advocacy documents all assume that depression is a public health problem of vast proportions, that relatively few sufferers receive appropriate professional treatment, and that more people need to take medication to overcome their suffering. Pharmaceutical companies have capitalized on reports of such large numbers of depressed people. Their ubiquitous advertisements emphasize symptoms such as sadness, loneliness, exhaustion, and anxiety that are widespread among people who are suffering from ordinary distress. These ads feature common situations such as family problems, difficulties at work, or the failure to accomplish desired goals, and they suggest that antidepressants are the most effective way to deal with these problems. The explosive growth in sales of antidepressant medications shows how effective their appeals have been.

It might seem as if defining normal suffering as a mental illness that requires professional treatment entails few risks and many benefits. Indeed, many antidepressant users do profit from the decreased distress and enhanced functioning that these medications can provide. Yet, antidepressants also entail a number of risks.

Hundreds of studies have been conducted about the effectiveness of antidepressant medications. Overall, they indicate that these drugs are more effective than placebo pills for persons with serious depression. However, for less than severe conditions the benefits from taking these medications often do not substantially exceed those of placebo. A comprehensive review of studies summarizes: "Although many trials do find antidepressants are superior to placebo, many do not, including some of the largest and most well-known landmark trials."[32] Studies that incorporate non-published as well as published research come to an even bleaker conclusion that their effectiveness is minimally greater than placebo effects in all but the most serious conditions.[33] This surprising outcome is due to the high proportions of people, often about 50%, with milder depressive conditions who respond positively to placebo. Perhaps the high placebo response rate indicates that what was being treated in the first place wasn't a disease but a distressing condition that can be overcome through obtaining basic support and caring.

Antidepressants are also not as benign as once believed. Many users experience side effects, such as sexual dysfunction, tremors, nausea, diarrhea, and headaches, among many others.[34] While the issue of physical and psychological dependence from long-term use is controversial, some experts have argued that many people suffer from serious psychological and physical consequences when they discontinue antidepressant use. When discontinuance is sudden, up to 25% of users can experience withdrawal problems.[35]

The medicalization of normal sadness also raises broader issues. Some amount of suffering is part of the human condition, and this part of life can be diminished when we call it a "disease."[36] In addition, although much suffering is an unavoidable aspect of being human, a considerable amount stems from oppressive and inequitable social arrangements and can best be addressed by changing these conditions. For example, providing more effective child-care arrangements for overworked parents might do more to effectively alleviate their distress than a pill can. Another important risk is that a misplaced emphasis on treating normal but unpleasant emotions can divert attention and transfer treatment resources away from persons with serious mental illnesses who are genuinely in need of them. We have been too ready to thoughtlessly medicalize normal distress without considering the profound negative resulting consequences.

SOCIAL ANXIETY DISORDER

Although depression is over-medicalized, there is no doubt that many people suffer from depressive mental disorders. Such disorders have been well-recognized since the earliest recorded medical histories. Other medicalized conditions, however, are far newer and indeed seem to have been created in order to treat them with pharmaceuticals. Social anxiety disorder (also called social phobia) is a prime example of this recent phenomenon.[37]

Social phobias are a condition that features extreme anxiety over situations where people are exposed to the scrutiny of others, such as when they must speak in public, have their performance evaluated, or attend social events that involve interacting with strangers. Their distress often leads them to avoid social situations where they fear the evaluations of others. Psychiatric diagnostic manuals did not mention this condition until 1980. When it first appeared, the manual noted that "the disorder is apparently relatively rare."[38] Initial studies of the disorder in the early 1980s indicated that about 1–2% of the population reported this condition. Yet, the most recent studies indicate that over 13%, or one of eight people, have had a social phobia at some point in their lives.[39] Indeed, by the early twenty-first century, social phobias were one of the two most common mental disorders. How did the number of people with this condition more than quintuple in such a short period of time?

Rising rates of social phobias are largely due to minor changes in how questions are asked about their symptoms. Having an unreasonably strong fear of public speaking is the most common symptom of the disorder. Just changing the wording of a question that asked about having extreme distress when "speaking in front of a group you know" to "speaking in front of a group" doubled the number of positive responses. Likewise, changing the criteria from having "a compelling desire to avoid" fear-inducing situations to having "marked distress" in these situations resulted in a sharp increase in the reported amount of social phobia.

The pharmaceutical industry quickly exploited the huge prevalence of a hitherto almost unknown disorder. In 1999 the antidepressant Paxil was approved for the specific treatment of social phobia. Its manufacturer, GlaxoSmithKline, mounted a huge advertising campaign, spending over $90 million on a barrage of print and television ads with the message "imagine being allergic to other people." These ads were just the small visible part of a gigantic public relations campaign by the firm Cohn & Wolfe aimed at fundamentally reshaping public perceptions of social anxiety from being shy and uneasy in social situations to having a mental disorder treatable with drugs.[40] Other aspects of the campaign involved placing stories in the news media, often using celebrity figures, psychiatric experts, and testimonies from members of consumer advocacy groups about the pervasiveness of and disabilities from social anxiety disorder. The immense public relations campaign was a huge success—Paxil became the highest selling antidepressant at the time, with sales of $3 billion a year. Social anxiety is now a common and well-recognized mental illness.

The creation of social anxiety disorder and the need to take medication to treat it shows how pharmaceutical companies can enlist advocacy groups and researchers and launch media campaigns that turn distressing but normal emotions such as shyness into widespread mental disorders. Some individuals, such as salespeople, teachers, or executives, whose jobs require them to speak before large audiences can truly benefit from getting professional help when they experience what is now called "social anxiety." Formerly shy people can now see themselves as having a mental disorder that has a pharmaceutical solution. For many, however, the risks of side effects, painful withdrawal effects, and long-term regimes of medication can outweigh any positive effects. If their condition disturbs them, anxious people might be better off with coaching or counseling rather than beginning potentially never-ending regimens of potent pharmaceuticals.

SEXUAL DYSFUNCTIONAL DISORDER

Medicalization does not just involve treating personal defects but has also expanded into the realm of enhancing social performance. The medicalization and attendant drug treatment of sexual behavior offers a prime example. The boom in the medicalization of sex began in 1998 when Pfizer put a new drug, Viagra, onto the market. Initially, the company thought that this drug would mostly attract older men with physical disabilities or illnesses that made it difficult for them to achieve sexual climaxes. They enlisted former United States senator, presidential candidate, and World War II veteran Robert Dole as their major spokesman for an extensive advertising campaign. It soon became clear, however, that Viagra had a much wider appeal to younger, sexually capable men who found that the drug could enhance their sexual performance. Subsequent advertising campaigns employing hyper-masculine sports figures targeted a much broader audience, deemphasized sexual dysfunctions, and asked if viewers were "not satisfied with your sex life?" Viagra and its close siblings Levetra and Cialis have generated huge sales for their makers, reaching $2.5 billion in 2004.

A widely publicized study that was published in the *Journal of the American Medical Association* (JAMA) in 1999 underlay pharmaceutical company confidence in the presence of a large market for their new products.[41] This study indicated that a remarkable 31% of men and 43% of women had "sexual dysfunctions." These figures stemmed from responses to seven questions asking whether respondents had a lack of interest in sex, had anxiety about sexual performance, had an inability to have an orgasm, found that sex was not pleasurable, and the like.

Such "symptoms," of course, can represent many conditions that are not sexual dysfunctions. Some might be reported by members of well-adjusted couples who no longer have a strong interest in having sex. Others might stem from having boring or inept sexual partners or from unsatisfactory or abusive relationships. Indeed, the study found that the best predictor of "sexual dysfunction" was low satisfaction with one's sexual partner. From a medicalized view, however, interpersonal problems are reinterpreted as medical symptoms that need a pharmaceutical remedy. Indeed, the authors of the *JAMA* study concluded that sexual dysfunction is a "public health" problem that calls for medical therapies, especially medications.

In fact, the findings of this study suggest that many people would be better advised to either change their relationships with their current partners or to find different partners instead of seeking medications that enhance sexual performance. Calling people with problems in their interpersonal relationships "sexually dysfunctional" might help the business of pharmaceutical companies, but it fundamentally mischaracterizes the nature of many of these problems.

These highly successful drugs for sexual dysfunction left a huge market untapped: women. The *JAMA* article with its 43% figure and the huge success of Viagra clearly indicated that a new drug for female sexual dysfunction could be the pharmaceutical industry's next blockbuster drug.[42] Numerous drug companies began to develop new products that might treat the presumed biological problem of female sexual dysfunction. The industry also organized a number of conferences for physicians that were based on the premise that female sexual problems were both medical dysfunctions and extremely widespread. Industry-sponsored experts received broad media coverage, especially in women's magazines and on daytime television talk shows.

The industry's efforts to develop testosterone or androgen supplements to treat female sexual dysfunction have not yet succeeded. No proposed drug exceeds the effectiveness of placebo. Worse, the developmental drugs have had alarming numbers of side effects, including increased hair growth, deepening of the voice, and increased risks of liver and heart disease.[43] The continuing efforts of pharmaceutical companies to medicalize women's bodies will test their power to reshape the nature of psychosocial problems into biological problems in need of chemical solutions.

Older age cohorts matured in an era when mental illness was equated with insanity and mental health treatment typically occurred in mental institutions. They thus often associate mental illness with highly stigmatizing conditions and resist the use of use of mental health treatment. Not surprisingly, surveys indicate that they have far lower rates of mental health service use than any other age group.[44]

Although the elderly are the most likely age group to resist defining their problems in mental health terms and using specialty mental health facilities, they are heavy consumers of medical services. Older persons are thus an extremely attractive target for drug companies because they combine a mostly untapped market of potential psychotropic drug use combined with extensive contact with the medical system. The Medicare Prescription Drug, Improvement, and Modernization Act that went into effect in 2006 provides especially generous pharmaceutical benefits to the elderly, making this group even more alluring to the pharmaceutical industry.

Since the 1990s extensive efforts have been made to get general physicians to recognize and treat depression among the elderly.[45] These efforts have generally succeeded and have led to a striking increase in diagnoses of depression in this age group.[46] Medicare data show that the proportion of elderly persons diagnosed with depression more than doubled between 1992 and 1998. Use of antidepressants in this population increased from 7.3% in 1992 to 12.5% in 1998, so that nearly one in eight elderly persons now use an antidepressant.

The growing rate of diagnoses of depression and of psychotropic drug use among the elderly has positive aspects. These medications can enhance functioning and quality of life, particularly after physical injuries and illnesses. Their rapid growth, however, also has associated risks. One is that elderly people often take many different kinds of medications and the potentially harmful interactions among them and antidepressant drugs are understudied. When proper care is not taken to ensure safe use, the elderly users can suffer from dangerous side effects from psychotropic medication. In addition, physicians often rely on inappropriate prescribing patterns for the elderly. Many prescribe benzodiazepines despite the adverse effects this type of medication has for many older persons.[47] In addition, physicians prescribe these medications for situations, such as normal grieving, where they can not only have negative side effects but also impede natural processes of bereavement.

Moreover, medications can be over-prescribed at the expense of other sorts of treatments. Responses to depression among the elderly typically involve the exclusive use of medication: 60.2% only receive antidepressants compared to 14.4% who only receive psychotherapy and to 25.5% who receive both.[48] Although rates of psychotherapy among the elderly are particularly low, many older persons might benefit more from general support than from medication. The growing medicalization of psychological problems among the elderly promises some benefits but also should proceed with caution because of its attendant risks.

THE RISKS OF MEDICALIZATION

The medicalization of social life has undoubtedly helped many people. The availability of effective medications is partly responsible for why far fewer people enter mental hospitals and far more live in the community than in past decades. Psychotropic drugs also allow many people to lead brighter lives and accomplish more than they would if they were not taking medications for their problems.

The benefits of medicalization, however, are often inflated. Although claims for the effectiveness of psychotropic medication are widely accepted, they are often overstated. While these drugs do help contain the worst symptoms of serious mental illnesses, they are not nearly as valuable for less severe conditions. Moreover, newer medications rarely are more effective than medications that were developed in earlier decades but are now off-patent and generically available. FDA approval does not require that some new medication be better than an older one but only that the medication exceed the benefits of a placebo in some trials. This means that many new drugs are not superior to the ones they succeed. They are, however, far more remunerative, and their average price is about three to four times higher than generic equivalents. Pharmaceutical companies and the patient advocacy groups they support relentlessly lobby for prescription coverage of new drugs that are under patent and therefore highly profitable. These drugs, at most, have marginal benefits but come at huge costs to third-party payers and, ultimately, to consumers.

If the benefits from psychotropic medications have been overestimated for many conditions, the opposite is true for their risks. Rates of negative side effects, including diminished sexual desire, increased somatic symptoms, and sleep problems as well as withdrawal problems from ceasing SSRIs and heightened suicidal potential, are underestimated.[49] Another serious question regards the near-total absence of data that addresses the impact of long-term use of psychotropic medications. Studies regarding effectiveness usually deal with periods of less than a year, and none show that long-term regimes of medication are safe. A comprehensive review by the British National Institute for Health and Clinical Excellence concludes: "Given doubts about their benefits and concern about their risks, current recommendations for prescribing antidepressants should be reconsidered."[50] This caution is particularly relevant for decisions regarding medicating children, whose brains are not completely developed.[51]

The medicalization of psychosocial problems also has economic implications. On the one hand, managed care insurance approaches, which generally rely on strategies that reduce health care expenditures by underwriting the least expensive possible treatments, are now a powerful social force promoting the use of medications.[52] Managed care encourages the use of general physicians, who almost always prescribe medications, instead of mental health specialists, who may be more likely to use alternatives. Because medication therapy takes considerably less practitioner and patient time than most psychotherapy, it is more amenable to the cost/benefit logic of managed care organizations. Most managed care plans, therefore, provide more generous benefits for pharmaceutical than for psychotherapeutic treatments.[53] Conversely, these plans usually place severe limits on payment for psychotherapies, which they view as less necessary and more wasteful than medication. Medication thus involves lower out-of-pocket costs for patients than psychotherapy does, which also influences patients themselves to prefer drug treatments.

On the other hand, public relations and advertising campaigns that target normal people and urge them to consider their conditions as diseases can be very costly to the medical system. The market for psychiatric drugs increased by over 600% between 1990 and 2000 and accounted for $19 billion in sales by the end of that decade.[54] Just two categories of medication accounted for 80% of the growth in psychiatric drug spending: the SSRIs (52%) and atypical antipsychotics (28%), both of which have been heavily promoted by pharmaceutical companies. Spending on the SSRIs increased from $3.4 billion in 1996 to $7.9 billion in 2001, an annual rate of 18.5%.[55] Over the last decade of the twentieth century, real spending for antidepressants rose from $137 million to $1.2 billion, while spending for stimulants rose from $12 million in 1991 to $158 million in 2001. Medicaid spending on psychotropic drugs experienced a remarkable growth from $0.6 billion to $6.7 billion over the same period.[56] Much of this spending is due to the demand for new antipsychotics, such as Risperdal and Zyprexa, that have not been shown to be more effective than older antipsychotic drugs but are far more profitable to their makers.

While the enormous growth in the use of psychotropic medications has had major implications for public and private funders, it is difficult to assess how this spending compares to the amount that would have been spent in the absence of these drugs. To the extent that ordinary emotions that would have gone untreated are now being medicated, medicalization has created rising costs in the health care system. In addition, much unnecessary cost accrues when brand-name drugs are prescribed instead of equivalent generics. Likewise, newer drugs that are far more expensive but not more effective than the drugs they replaced are responsible for a substantial amount of unnecessary expense.

THE MEDICALIZATION SYNDROME

It is becoming increasingly clear that the enormous rise in apparent mental illness and the use of drugs to treat it does not result from medicine's greater ability to identify and treat diseases that went unrecognized in the past.[57] Medicalization has created many of the conditions that it claims to treat.[58] Some of these conditions, such as pediatric bipolar disorder or social phobia, barely existed until recently. Others, including ADHD, Major Depressive Disorder, and sexual dysfunction, were well-recognized disorders, but medicalization has greatly broadened the criteria that define them.

The drug industry has become a powerful force that shapes the boundaries between the normal and the pathological. Direct-to-consumer advertising does not simply attempt to sell particular products but strives to reshape consumers' understanding of their problems into conditions that should be treated by medications. Medicalization involves far more than specific treatments but entails an entire worldview about the nature, cause, and remedy for psychosocial problems. For example, a woman having difficulties with her husband who views an ad that claims an antidepressant drug can relieve her sadness, anxiety, and fatigue is encouraged to see her distress as a mental disease that causes, rather than results from, disturbances in family life. Constant reminders to screen every possible discomfort for signs of disease do not seem to be the optimal way of promoting mental health.

Pharmaceutical companies have successfully medicalized psychosocial problems that in the past were perceived as having little in common with disease. This is most apparent during childhood, where ADHD, bipolar disorder, and depression, among many other conditions, now seem to be rampant where they were virtually unknown just a few years ago. Adults too now seem to suffer from depression, social phobia, adult attention deficit disorder, and sexual dysfunction—not to mention panic attacks, post-traumatic stress disorder, eating disorders, multiple personality disorders, and many other disorders—at far higher rates than ever before. Even the elderly, who once made strenuous efforts to avoid seeing their problems through a psychiatric lens, take psychotropic medications in ever-growing numbers.

The influence of pharmaceutical companies extends well beyond overt advertising to subsidizing those advocacy groups that promote the view that chemical deficiencies cause mental illness, placing stories featuring celebrities with particular kinds of mental illnesses in the news media, sponsoring continuing education seminars for physicians, funding psychiatric research, and supporting public service messages, Internet self-help sites, and mental health awareness days. The relentless message stemming from these efforts is that mental illnesses are not ordinary psychosocial problems but are real diseases that require chemical solutions. Media campaigns have fundamentally changed the ways that people understand and express their experiences as well as the ways that physicians have come to treat these experiences.

A new frontier of medicalization lies in convincing people who might not even have any symptoms at all that they are "at risk" for developing a psychiatric illness and should take medication in order to prevent some condition from actually arising.[59] Far more people might have some genetic marker that might elevate their chances of developing a mental illness than will ever actually become mentally ill. For example, up to two-thirds of the population has a gene that is purportedly connected with elevated rates of depression.[60] Because people who are genetically "at risk" for such episodes as well as people who have actually suffered a depressive episode become candidates for drug interventions, the market for products that might prevent some condition from arising is potentially huge. A new "at-risk" phenotype of non-symptomatic individuals who nonetheless consume genetically tailored psychotropic drugs for long periods of time could be the next stage of a medicalized society.

Finally, medicalization has entailed the assumption that drugs are the treatment of choice for numerous psychosocial problems. Definitions of normality have involved progressively lowered thresholds for medical interventions in recent years. Prescribing pills can send messages that issues such as unfulfilling marriages, poor parenting, inadequate finances, and the like are easily remedied through pharmaceuticals. Current health policy has become overly reliant on using medical remedies for concerns that often can be addressed through alternative social policies. Enhancing parenting skills, investing in childhood development programs, and improving child-care resources might be more effective responses to childhood behavioral problems than pharmaceutical treatments. Promoting healthy lifestyles and reducing socioeconomic inequality, workplace pressures, and family demands could counteract the circumstances that lead people to want to use pills to alter their distressing psychological conditions in the first place. Changes in social arrangements might lead to more improvement in mental health than calling people ill and prescribing pills to remedy their conditions.

NOTES

1   Peter Conrad, *The Medicalization of Society: On the Transformation of Human Conditions into Medical Disorders* (Baltimore: Johns Hopkins University Press, 2007).

2   Mark Olfson et al., "National Trends in the Treatment of Attention Deficit Hyperactivity Disorder," *American Journal of Psychiatry* 160 (2003): 1071–77.

3   Susanna N. Visser, Catherine Lesesne, and Ruth Perou, "National Estimates and Factors Associated With Medication Treatment for Childhood Attention-Deficit/Hyperactivity Disorder," *Pediatrics* 119, supp. 1 (2007): S99–S106.

4 Samuel H. Zuvekas, Benedetto Vitiello, and Grayson S. Norquist, "Recent Trends in Stimulant Medication Use Among U.S. Children," *American Journal of Psychiatry* 163 (2006): 579–85.

5 Alison E. Cuellar and Sara Markowitz, "Medicaid Policy Changes in Mental Health Care and Their Effect on Mental Health Services," *Health Economics, Policy and Law* 2 (2007): 23–49.

6 Lawrence H. Diller, *The Last Normal Child* (Westport, CT: Praeger, 2006).

7 American Psychiatric Association, *Diagnostic and Statistical Manual of Mental Disorders*, 4th ed., text revision (Washington, DC: American Psychiatric Association, 2000).

8 Diller, *The Last Normal Child*.

9 Zuvekas et al., "Recent Trends in Stimulant Medication."

10 Olfson et al., "National Trends in the Treatment of Attention Deficit."

11 U.S. Department of Health and Human Services, *Mental Health, United States 2004* (Washington, DC: U.S. Government Printing Office, 2007).

12 Cindy Thomas et al., "Trends in the Use of Psychotropic Medications among Adolescents, 1994–2001," *Psychiatric Services* 57 (2006): 63–69.

13 Julie M. Zito et al., "Psychotropic Practice Patterns for Youth," *Archives of Pediatric and Adolescent Medicine* 157 (2003): 17–25.

14 Jeffrey Bridge et al., "Clinical Response and Risk for Reported Suicidal Ideation and Suicide Attempts in Pediatric Antidepressant Treatment: A Meta-Analysis of Randomized Controlled Trials," *Journal of the American Medical Association* 297 (2007): 1683–96.

15 Dean Fergusson et al., "Association between Suicide Attempts and Selective Serotonin Reuptake Inhibitors: Systematic Review of Randomised Controlled Trials," *British Medical Journal* 330 (2005): 396–99.

16 Mark Olfson, Steven C. Marcus, and David Shaffer, "Antidepressant Drug Therapy and Suicide in Severely Depressed Children and Adults," *Archives of General Psychiatry* 63 (2006): 865–72.

17 National Institute of Mental Health, "Antidepressant Medications for Children and Adolescents: Information for Parents and Caregivers," http://www.nimh.nih.gov/health/topics/child-and-adolescent-mental-health/antidepressant-medications-for-children-and-adolescents-information-for-parents-and-caregivers.shtml.

18 Eliot Marshall, "Buried Data Can Be Hazardous To a Company's Health," *Science* 304 (2004): 1576–77.

19 Mark Olfson et al., "National Trends in the Outpatient Treatment of Children and Adolescents With Antipsychotic Drugs," *Archives of General Psychiatry* 63 (2006): 679–85.

20 Olfson et al., "National Trends in the Outpatient Treatment."

21 Carmen Moreno et al., "National Trends in the Outpatient Diagnosis and Treatment of Bipolar Disorder in Youth," *Archives of General Psychiatry* 64 (2007): 1032–39.

22 Jerome Groopman, "What's Normal?: The Difficulty of Diagnosing Bipolar Disorder in Children," *New Yorker*, April 9, 2007.

23 Benjamin G. Druss et al., "Listening to Generic Prozac: Winners, Losers, and Sideliners," *Health Affairs* 23 (2004): 210–16.

24 Gardiner Harris and Benedict Carey, "Researchers Fail to Reveal Full Drug Pay," *New York Times*, June 8, 2008.

25 New Freedom Commission on Mental Health, *Achieving the Promise: Transforming Mental Health Care in America* (Rockville, MD: U.S. Department of Health and Human Services, 2003).

26 David Healy, *Let Them Eat Prozac* (New York: New York University Press, 2004).

27 Olfson et al., "National Trends in the Treatment of Attention Deficit."

28 Ronald C. Kessler et al., "Prevalence, Severity, and Comorbidity of 12-Month DSM-IV Disorders in the National Comorbidity Survey Replication," *Archives of General Psychiatry* 62 (2005): 617–27.

29 Nikolas Rose, "Disorders Without Borders? The Expanding Scope of Psychiatric Practice," *Biosocieties* 1 (2006): 465–84.

30 Kessler et al., "Prevalence, Severity, and Comorbidity."

31 Allan V. Horwitz and Jerome C. Wakefield, *The Loss of Sadness* (New York: Oxford University Press, 2007).

32 Joanna Moncrieff and Irving Kirsch, "Efficacy of Antidepressants in Adults," *British Medical Journal* 331 (2005): 155–59.

33 Irving Kirsch et al., "Initial Severity and Antidepressant Benefits: A Meta-Analysis of Data Submitted to the Food and Drug Administration," *PLoS Medicine* 5, no. 2 (2008): e45.

34 Joseph Glenmullen, *Prozac Backlash* (New York: Simon & Schuster, 2000).

35 Charles Medawar and Anita Hardon, *Medicines Out of Control? Antidepressants and the Conspiracy of Goodwill* (Amsterdam: Aksant, 2004).

36 Carl Elliott, *Better than Well: American Medicine Meets the American Dream* (New York: Norton, 2003).

37 Christopher Lane, *Shyness: How Normal Behavior Became a Sickness* (New Haven: Yale University Press, 2007).

38 American Psychiatric Association, *Diagnostic and Statistical Manual of Mental Disorders*, 3rd edition (Washington, DC: American Psychiatric Association, 1980).

39 William Magee et al., "Agoraphobia, Simple Phobia, and Social Phobia in the National Comorbidity Survey," *Archives of General Psychiatry* 53 (1996): 159–68.

40 Ray Moynihan and Alan Cassells, *Selling Sickness: How the World's Biggest Pharmaceutical Companies Are Turning Us All into Patients* (New York: Nation Books, 2005).

41 Edward O. Laumann, Anthony Paik, and Raymond C. Rosen, "Sexual Dysfunction in the United States: Prevalence and Predictors," *Journal of the American Medical Association* 281 (1999): 537–44.

42 Heather Hartley, "The 'Pinking' of Viagra Culture: Drug Industry Efforts to Create and Repackage Sex Drugs for Women," *Sexualities* 9 (2006): 363–78.

43 Heather Hartley, "Big Pharma in our Bedrooms: An Analysis of the Medicalization of Women's Sexual Problems," *Advances in Gender Research* 7 (2003): 89–129.

44 Philip S. Wang et al., "Twelve-Month Use of Mental Health Services in the United States," *Archives of General Psychiatry* 62 (2005): 629–40.

45 B. D. Lebowitz et al., "Diagnosis and Treatment of Depression in Late Life: Consensus Statement Update," *Journal of the American Medical Association* 278 (1997): 1186–90.

46 Stephen Crystal et al., "Diagnosis and Treatment of Depression in the Elderly Medicare Population: Predictors, Disparities, and Trends," *Journal of the American Geriatric Society* 51 (2003): 1718–28.

47 Joan M. Cook et al., "Physicians' Perspectives on Prescribing Benzodiazepines for Older Adults," *Journal of General Internal Medicine* 22 (2007): 303–7.

48 Crystal et al., "Diagnosis and Treatment of Depression."

49 Medawar and Hardon, *Medicines Out of Control*; Healy, *Let Them Eat Prozac.*

50 Moncrieff and Kirsch, "Efficacy of Antidepressants in Adults," 158.

51 James F. Leckman and Robert A. King, "A Developmental Perspective on the Controversy Surrounding the Use of SSRIs to Treat Pediatric Depression," *American Journal of Psychiatry* 164 (2007): 1304–5.

52 David Mechanic, *Mental Health and Social Policy: Beyond Managed Care* (Boston: Allyn & Bacon, 2007).

53 David M. Cutler, *Your Money or Your Life: Strong Medicine for America's Health Care System* (New York: Oxford University Press, 2004).

54 Rose, "Disorders Without Borders?"

55 Samuel H. Zuvekas, "Prescription Drugs and the Changing Patterns of Treatment for Mental Disorders, 1996–2001," *Health Affairs* 24 (2005): 195–205.

56 Cuellar and Markowitz, "Medicaid Policy Changes."

57 Conrad, *The Medicalization of Society.*

58 Rose, "Disorders Without Borders?"

59 Nikolas Rose, *The Politics of Life Itself* (Princeton: Princeton University Press, 2007).

60 Avshalom Caspi et al., "Influence of Life Stress on Depression: Moderation by a Polymorphism in the 5-HTT Gene," *Science* 301 (2003): 386–89.

CHAPTER FIVE

Medicalization and Risk Scares: The Case of Menopause and HRT

CHERYL STULTS AND PETER CONRAD

Medicalization describes a process by which nonmedical problems become defined and treated as medical problems, usually in terms of illnesses or disorders.[1] Many social scientists have been critical of medicalization, especially the "over-medicalization" of society, emphasizing its potential for adverse social and medical consequences. The engines behind medicalization have shifted in recent decades from medical professionals and social movements like Alcoholics Anonymous and the definition of alcoholism and the movements promoting the acceptance of post traumatic stress disorder (PTSD) to the pharmaceutical industry and consumers.[2] Pharmaceutical companies play a central role in the medicalization process by developing medications for a life problem and promoting its medicalization and treatment. But there have been numerous cases when the medications being promoted are found to have adverse effects and increase the risk for patients. When these adverse effects become known to the public, we can say a "risk scare" takes place. In this chapter, we examine the dynamics of the development of risk scares and the implications for patients/consumers and regulatory agencies as well as for the process of medicalization.

A risk scare generally occurs when new—and sometimes controversial—research findings or regulatory actions associate an existing product or procedure with an unexpected increased risk of illness or death and these findings are widely publicized by the media. The scare is usually triggered by the publication of medical or scientific studies that indicate that a specific medical treatment once thought to be beneficial now shows serious adverse or harmful effects. The media reports these studies and disseminates stories of the "danger" of the treatment, frequently as lead stories on nightly news broadcasts, on the front page of newspapers, and as cover stories in magazines. The media simplifies the study results and transmits portions of the findings that generate and create confusion and often panic not only to the consumers of the treatment but also to those who prescribe it. A frequent result of this is a dramatic decrease in product use.

In recent years, we have seen major risk scares in the media about Cox-2 inhibitors for pain (Vioxx and Celebrex) increasing risk of heart attacks or stroke, and selective serotonin reuptake inhibitors (SSRIs) increasing the risk of suicide behavior in adolescents. Historically, there have been many other risk scares, including scares about silicone breast implants and Fen-Phen for weight loss. In this chapter, we examine in detail the case of menopause and hormone replacement therapy (HRT), which affected millions of women and involved several risk scares. We begin with a brief review of how menopause, a natural life event, became a treatable disorder.

MENOPAUSE AND HORMONE REPLACEMENT THERAPY

Menopause has been medicalized since the 1930s and 1940s as a "deficiency disease,"[3] often with the recommendation of treatment with hormone replacement therapy (HRT). This is a classic case of taking a normal life course event and pathologizing it as a disorder or risk needing medical intervention. Clearly menopause creates physical "discomforts" but is not a life-threatening risk in and of itself to women's health. The medicalization of menopause began with the pharmaceutical development and production of both natural and synthetic estrogens and a series of medical publications validating their existence.[4] The first synthetic estrogen was created in 1938, but official approval from the Food and Drug Administration (FDA) did not occur until 1942, when Premarin, manufactured by Ayerst Laboratories (now known as Wyeth), was approved for the treatment of menopausal symptoms, including hot flashes, night sweats, and vaginal dryness.[5] Coinciding with the development and production of synthetic estrogen, a series of medical publications discussing menopause and its accompanying symptoms appeared from 1938 to 1941, further legitimizing this treatment.[6] One physician in a 1940s issue of the *American Journal of Obstetrics and Gynecology* noted that the verdict was "practically unanimous" on the efficacy of synthetic estrogen for the treatment of menopause.[7]

There is a long history of the medicalization of women's bodies and "troubles," including the late nineteenth century use of "hysteria" as a general diagnosis for the maladies of women and the twentieth century treatment of menopause.[8] By midcentury, physicians in association with the pharmaceutical industry were active in medicalizing women's problems. Doctors, such as gynecologist Robert A. Wilson, acted as moral entrepreneurs advocating HRT for their patients. Dr. Wilson's 1966 book *Feminine Forever* furthered the medicalization of menopause by greatly influencing public perceptions that estrogen therapy could combat the "disease" of menopause and help keep women "feminine forever." He claimed menopausal women were "living decay" who could be rescued from "being condemned to witness the death of their womanhood" through estrogen therapy.[9] His views were primarily based upon observations of his menopausal patients who had taken estrogen. The pharmaceutical industry significantly supported Wilson's research by donating $1.3 million in grants to the Wilson Foundation in 1963, with the primary purpose of promoting estrogen.[10]

Between 1950 and 1970, the pharmaceutical industry took a direct role in the promotion of HRT through advertisements to physicians. The advertisements appeared in medical journals, including the prestigious *Journal of the American Medical Association* (JAMA). Many advertisements during the 1960s featured a woman over 40 in black and white, looking sad and dejected while facing her physician—implying that the woman could become happy again through the help of her doctor prescribing her estrogen.[11] Later advertisements in the 1960s and 1970s urged physicians to "give back something she had lost," while depicting a lonely, melancholic woman staring into space (see figure 5.1).[12] These pharmaceutical advertisements promoted and reinforced the notion of menopause as a deficiency disease needing treatment with HRT.

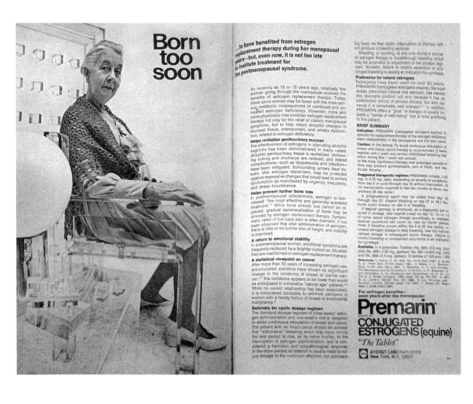

Figure 5.1   1969 HRT advertisement: "Born too soon...to have benefited from
estrogen replacement therapy during her menopausal years—but, even now,
it is not too late to institute treatment for the postmenopausal syndrome."

[Source: *Journal of the American Medical Association* 210, no. 1 (1969): 70–71]

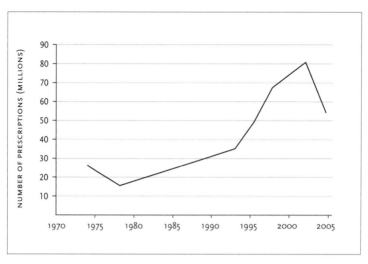

Figure 5.2   Approximate number of oral HRT prescriptions (estrogen and estrogen + progestin) before and after risk scares, 1974–2005

[Source: authors, based on data compiled from Adam L. Hersh, Marcia L. Stefanick, and Randall S. Stafford, "National Use of Postmenopausal Hormone Therapy: Annual Trends and Responses to Recent Evidence," *Jouranl of the American Medical Association* 291, no. 1 (2004): 47–53; and Sumit R. Majumdar, Elizabeth A. Almasi, and Randall S. Stafford, "Promotion and Prescribing of Hormone Replacement Therapy After Report of Harm by the Women's Health Initiative," *Journal of the American Medical Association* 292, no. 16 (2004): 1983–88]

In response to advice from their physicians and books like *Feminine Forever*, American women embraced HRT. Although there was recurrent criticism about its potential risks, over the years HRT continued to be a major medical treatment for menopause. By 1975, estrogen was the fifth most frequently prescribed drug in the United States, with 26–30 million prescriptions annually (see figure 5.2).[13]

INCREASED RISKS FOR PATIENTS

In the context of the widespread utilization of HRT, physicians discovered adverse medical problems. As early as 1947, a Columbia University oncologist, Saul Gusberg, suggested that HRT increased the risk of endometrial (uterine) cancer. These findings, however, were not widely publicized. One possible reason was HRT's effectiveness in providing relief from the main menopausal symptoms of hot flashes and night sweats with the ease of taking a pill and at relatively low cost trumped the potential disadvantages. Physicians at the time believed that the risk shown in this one study did not outweigh the benefits of estrogen. In 1975, the *New England Journal of Medicine* published two independent studies reporting that women on HRT had a four- to twentyfold increased risk of uterine cancer. Other studies with similar results followed, creating apprehension among women and their physicians. These findings and their publicizing by the media triggered the first HRT risk scare.

In the wake of these reports, governmental organizations began to produce summary statements aimed at physicians regarding the prescription of estrogen. The FDA responded to the scare by holding two years of public hearings before issuing the July 1977 ruling that mandated a patient package insert for estrogens that noted the risk of adverse events like endometrial cancer.[14] The National Institute on Aging later recommended in 1979: "ERT [estrogen replacement therapy] is only effective in the treatment of hot flashes and vaginal atrophy, and if used at all, should be administered on a cyclical basis (three weeks of estrogen, one week off) at the lowest dose for the shortest possible time."[15] American women and their physicians responded to this risk scare with a dramatic 40% decrease in the number of prescriptions of HRT—from 26.7 million in 1975 to 16 million in 1978 (see figure 5.2).[16] For many women in the late 1970s, the risks of HRT had exceeded its benefits. Still, drug company promotion persuaded physicians to write 16 million prescriptions for their patients, despite the publicized risks. The FDA noted in 1978 that, despite a major decline, menopausal estrogens remained "grossly overused" given the risk of endometrial cancer and recommended that they be used for "severe" menopausal symptoms, which not all menopausal women experience.[17]

COUNTERCLAIMS OF RISK REDUCTION

Drug companies searched for a "safer" alternative. Such an alternative appeared later in the 1980s, when the combination of estrogen with progestin was shown to eliminate the excess risk of uterine cancer in women who still had their uterus.[18] In 1995, estrogen and progestin were combined into a single pill, Prempro, that could be taken once a day. This alternative expanded the market for pharmaceutical companies since now women who had had a hysterectomy could "safely" take estrogen alone, while women with a uterus could "safely" take the combination.

With the creation of the combination HRT came a shift in the promotion of estrogens. Up to this time, the recommendation for using HRT consisted only of relief of menopausal symptoms like hot flashes, night sweats, and vaginal dryness. But, fueled by the results of some clinical studies suggesting that the new estrogen pills could reduce risk of some serious diseases, the new marketing focus shifted to reducing the risk of developing other disorders, particularly heart disease, osteoporosis, Alzheimer's, and breast cancer. These newfound benefits for prevention were promoted by both physicians and the pharmaceutical industry. Medical and scientific journals published articles that posited estrogen protects women against heart disease and the increased risk of osteoporosis after menopause.[19] At this time, it appeared that the lower levels of estrogen placed women at an increased risk of heart disease and osteoporosis, and it seemed "natural" to replace the estrogen they had lost with HRT. While increased risk of heart disease and osteoporosis occurs with aging in general, physicians at the time focused only on menopause since women's bodies were under close medical scrutiny. The Nurses' Health Study (NHS) provided the largest amount of data supporting this link between women and heart disease. More important, multiple observational studies suggested that HRT engendered a 50% reduction in coronary artery disease, the leading cause of death in American women. Two clinical trials in the late 1980s and early 1990s demonstrated a substantial reduction in osteoporosis with HRT.[20] During this time, the overall conception of HRT was clearly in a new stage, as an intervention to reduce the *risk* of other serious and deadly diseases instead of just a treatment to appease bothersome menopausal symptoms.

Pharmaceutical company advertising had changed following the 1975 risk scare. The late 1970s ads, which appeared in top medical journals aimed at physicians, had a goal of expanding the range of individuals who might need HRT: no longer just older working women and homemakers, but now elegant socialites became market targets. Ads in the 1980s and 1990s depicted women smiling, dancing, and looking for romance, implying that a good life could be attained through estrogen. Beginning in the early 1980s advertisements began to focus on the treatment of osteoporosis with estrogen, noting that "ten million women might benefit (see figure 5.3)."[21] Thus, pharmaceutical advertising for physicians refocused on HRT as a risk preventive drug for women.

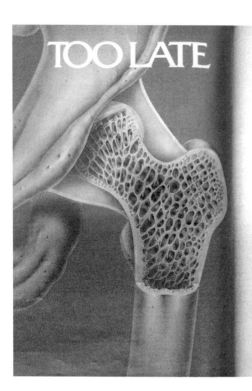

Figure 5.3   1985 HRT advertisement: "Too Late. Improve the Outlook for Osteoporosis."

[Source: *Journal of the American Medical Association* 254, no. 13 (1985): 1742–43]

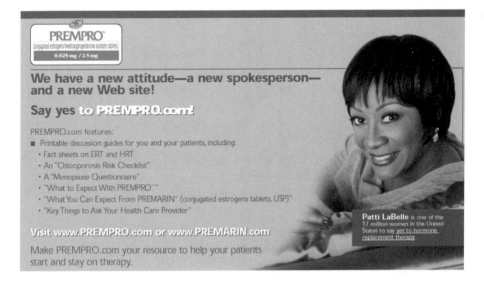

Figure 5.4   2002 HRT advertisement featuring Patti LaBelle

[Source: http://www.edocktor.com/drennan/prempro.pdf (accessed June 16, 2008)]

Advertising changed dramatically in 1997 with the new FDA regulations that allowed for direct-to-consumer advertising (DTCA) on television, reinvigorating the medicalization of menopause. New regulations allowed advertisers to shorten the potentially long lists of risks, provided they offer some way for the consumer to access the information (for example, a Web site, referenced advertisement, or phone number).[22] This resulted in an increased number of advertisements for HRT, with a two-pronged marketing strategy—treating the "deficiency disease" along with lowering risk for other diseases. In 2002 alone, Wyeth spent more than $38 million on DTCA for its combination estrogen and progestin drug, Prempro.[23] These ads portrayed women as sexy and attractive, using older spokeswomen such as Lauren Hutton and Patti LaBelle to promote the benefits of HRT (see figure 5.4).[24] These ads implied that taking estrogen would help women look and feel as sexy as these celebrities, reviving the "feminine forever" theme, but this time with reduced risk.

Medical research continued to tout risk benefits, amplified enormously by pharmaceutical promotion, leading to soaring prescription rates for HRT. By 2000 Premarin became the most frequently prescribed brand-name drug in the United States.[25] With the 1975 risk scare now a distant memory, more than 15 million women—estimated at nearly 42% of all women aged 50 to 74 years—were using estrogen in 2001, resulting in 80.8 million prescriptions that year (see figure 5.2).[26]

PATIENT RISK INCREASED, NOT REDUCED

To further investigate the claims concerning the preventative benefits of HRT, the National Institutes of Health (NIH) sponsored an eight-year, large-scale, randomized double-blind, placebo-controlled clinical trial, the current "gold standard" for medical research. So strong was the belief that the trial would confirm a large reduction in coronary heart disease incidence, that one physician suggested it was "unethical to leave volunteers on the placebos for the full eight and a half years of the trial. At some point, they'll have to stop the study and offer hormones to everyone."[27]

The Women's Health Initiative (WHI), as the trial was called, focused on 16,600 healthy, postmenopausal women aged 50–79, randomized to receive a formulation of estrogen (the formulation depended on whether they had had a hysterectomy) or a placebo. Originally planned for 8.5 years, in July 2002 the estrogen/progestin arm unexpectedly terminated after 5.2 years *when the cumulative risks of severe adverse outcomes outweighed the benefits.* The results, published in the July 2002 issue of *JAMA*, noted an *increased risk* for coronary heart disease, breast cancer, stroke, and venous thromboembolism (blood clots), which greatly outweighed the protective benefits for osteoporosis and colon cancer.[28]

These WHI findings were generally presented in two formats — as percentages of risk or rates of occurrence. The news media tended to use percentages to heighten the perception of risks for women, such as noting a 29% increased risk of heart disease for those taking estrogen/progestin. Pharmaceutical companies and some physicians tended to minimize the risks by using rates of occurrence, such as an additional four cases of heart disease for every 10,000 women using HRT. By framing the risks in these ways, each group maximized the results to their own benefit: the media reinforced the sense of panic experienced by women, while the pharmaceutical industry and some physicians presented the risks as less significant thereby encouraging the continuance of HRT. Among the roughly 15 million American women who took HRT in 2001, an estimated 14,500 adverse events could be attributed to HRT that year.[29]

In the years following the initial publication of their findings, WHI investigators reported additional results from the study that further emphasized the unfavorable risk-benefit ratio of HRT, heightening the risk scare for women and their physicians. HRT not only induced more breast cancers than placebo, but these breast cancers were also more advanced and less easily detected by mammograms.[30] Whereas previous observational data suggested that HRT might improve cognitive function in older women, a sub-study of the WHI, the Women's Health Initiative Memory Study (WHIMS), found that HRT actually doubled the risk of Alzheimer's disease and other dementias. Moreover, HRT did not improve a general sense of well-being or quality of life for asymptomatic women who were not experiencing vasomotor symptoms, such as hot flashes. Instead, general health, physical functioning, role limitations, bodily pain, energy and fatigue, social functioning, and mental health were all unchanged with HRT as compared to placebo.[31] In short, not only did HRT fail to reduce risk, it significantly increased the risk of serious diseases. By the end of 2003, annual prescription rates for oral HRT had fallen from 80.2 million in 2001 to 55.7 million.[32]

As it turned out, the section of the WHI project that continued studying estrogen alone after July 2002 also terminated one year early in 2004, this time due to an increased risk of stroke.[33] Similar to the estrogen and progestin study, the risk of stroke increased with eight additional cases for every 10,000 women. While a benefit of decreased fractures also was noted in this study, the investigators reported "no effect"—neither an increase nor a decrease—on coronary heart disease and breast cancer. The investigators debated whether to alert patients to the risk of stroke and continue the study but concluded that "an increased risk of stroke is not acceptable in healthy women in a research study," especially since there was no benefit of a risk reduction of coronary heart disease. This was an unusual move, since none of the predefined stopping barriers for the trial were crossed; given the reaction to the estrogen/progestin arm of the WHI in July 2002, however, the investigators felt it best to avoid any further harm.

In 2003 the *Lancet* published results of a study that reinforced the risk scare.[34] This study, conducted with one million women in the United Kingdom, found that women taking *any kind of hormone replacement therapy*, regardless of the type (e.g., either estrogen or estrogen/progestin), had an increased risk of breast cancer. More specifically, the study demonstrated that combined estrogen and progestin HRT increased breast cancer risk fourfold, rates similar to those seen with HRT in the WHI study.

These studies received much media and public attention in 2002 and 2003, with hundreds of newspaper articles and thousands of television and radio reports. While the WHI findings triggered a major risk scare, it is interesting to note an earlier study that reported similar adverse outcomes was not widely publicized by the media, apparently due to the limits of the study population. In 1998, the Heart and Estrogen/Progestin Replacement Study (HERS) found an increase in both heart attack and stroke after the first year of HRT, findings contradictory to the previously reported benefits.[35] However, because the results of this study were observational and not a randomized clinical trial (the current "gold standard" of research), the findings were not widely publicized by the media and did not create a risk scare. Most physicians continued to accept that HRT would reduce the risk of coronary heart disease in healthy women since the American Heart Association only provided a warning for a select group of women—those with coronary artery disease (CAD) — rather than all HRT users. In retrospect, these findings could have shown women with CAD to be the canaries in the coal mine. But these HRT "canaries" weren't recognized until publication of the WHI results four years later. Until the 2002 risk scare, the risks of HRT were not of great concern to the public. But while women and physicians during the period of 1995–2002 believed that HRT was reducing their risks of chronic illnesses and the pharmaceutical companies aggressively promoted this view in their marketing, the tragic irony was that the assumed beneficial drug actually increased the risks for the illnesses it was purporting to protect against.

MEDIA AMPLIFICATION AND RISK SCARE RESPONSES

A key element to a risk scare is a drug's risks becoming widely publicized. News of the unexpected, adverse consequences of HRT reported in the randomized clinical trials and other studies was rapidly disseminated not only to physicians and other health care providers but also to the public at large. In just the first month following the July 2002 publication, there were more than 400 newspaper stories and 2,500 television/radio reports.[36] One researcher examined articles from the top five circulating newspapers from 2002 to 2003 and found only 3% contained accurate information about the risks. Additionally, the coverage of HRT was overwhelmingly negative, "vilifying" the pharmaceutical companies and physicians.[37] Some small studies suggested that the overall media coverage resulted in a reported 30–50% decrease in HRT use.[38] In an editorial in the *Annals of Internal Medicine,* Lisa Schwartz and Steven Woloshin hypothesize that most of this decrease is due to the media's rapid dissemination of the findings.[39] Another study, by Jennifer Haas and others, found that of twenty-two newspapers in seven representative areas of the United States, 83% of the articles published in July 2002 included coverage of the potential harmful effects of HRT.[40] The authors found that, on average, women were exposed to fewer than one article a day detailing the harmful effects of HRT. However, when the researchers divided their findings by region, they determined that women in the San Francisco Bay area were exposed to HRT coverage at a rate of three articles per day. Examining data about each area, they found that women exposed to a greater number of articles had higher rates of termination of HRT. Thus, while others stated that overall media coverage led to the HRT decline, this study suggested that greater rates of media coverage correlated to greater declines in HRT use.

Although the findings are suggestive, a major limitation of this study is that the authors do not know if any individual woman who chose to terminate HRT actually read any articles; they just took the generalized data for each geographical area and connected it with the newspaper media coverage for that area. It is difficult from these data to attribute cause to media exposure. But it seems clear that while the medical findings triggered the risk scare, the news media were key in disseminating the findings and amplifying the public's concern about HRT and its newly discovered risks.

REGULATORY AND PROFESSIONAL WARNINGS

Nearly one month after the publication of the July 2002 article from the WHI estrogen and progestin trial, the Food and Drug Administration released a press statement about the findings.[41] After briefly stating the increased risks, the FDA reiterated that estrogens had not been approved for coronary heart disease or any other cardio-protective benefit or for cognitive benefits and that physicians should not prescribe the drug for these purposes. The only FDA-approved uses for estrogens are treatment of "moderate to severe" vasomotor symptoms, treatment of vulvar and vaginal atrophy, and prevention of osteoporosis. The FDA also suggested that women consult their physicians regarding the findings and that while each decision is "highly individualized" according to risks and benefits, women should seek the lowest dose for the shortest time possible. Since other preventive treatments were available for osteoporosis, the FDA recommended that women should consider these options first and that HRT be given to those who cannot use the non-estrogen options. With these recommendations, the FDA attempted to take a cautious course regarding the use of HRT. While not fully condemning the usage of HRT for osteoporosis, the FDA advised women and physicians to consider other treatment modalities first before considering estrogen, thus not further amplifying the risks.

In addition to these recommendations, the FDA also mandated changes in the labeling of estrogens and estrogen plus progestin to note the increased risks identified in the WHI studies. The new "black box" warning (the highest FDA warning short of banning the drug) emphasized the increased risks of myocardial infarction, breast cancer, stroke, and venous thromboembolism and stated that the drug should not be used to prevent coronary heart disease. Additional treatment clarifications and guidelines were also provided.

Following the FDA, major medical organizations (including the North American Menopause Society and the American College of Obstetrics and Gynecology) also shifted their position on the use of HRT.[42] Similar to the FDA recommendations, they suggested that HRT should be used only to treat women with severe menopausal symptoms in as small a dose and for as short a time possible, "consistent with treatment goals and risks for individual women." There was no consensus as to the particular dose or the specific length of time for HRT to be prescribed. These organizations also suggested that women currently taking HRT should consider discontinuing the medication after consultation with their physicians. They also recommended that while HRT does reduce the risk for postmenopausal osteoporotic fractures, alternative therapies are available and should be considered. Their overall conclusion was that there is no role for HRT in the prevention of chronic disease.

PHARMACEUTICAL COMPANY RESPONSE

In contrast to the FDA, pharmaceutical companies took a more nuanced approach of damage control when acknowledging the newfound risks of HRT. While they attempted to present a face of corporate responsibility to consumers, the clear goal was to maintain a market for their HRT drug. On September 4, 2002, nearly two months after the initial WHI results, Wyeth issued a press statement announcing an update to their estrogen package inserts due to the findings of the WHI study.[43] Wyeth mailed letters to physicians informing them of the change, restating the major points made by the FDA. Wyeth's vice president felt that this new information would assist physicians "in assessing each patient's individual risks and treatment goals."[44] Wyeth would also "continue to work closely with the medical community and regulatory authorities to further refine its product labels for all of its postmenopausal hormone therapies, regardless of the estrogen or progestin used." Since 2002, Wyeth has subsequently commented on findings—both beneficial and adverse—that have been published in the major medical journals. Their most recent statement, in June 2007, indicated that "Wyeth continues to support the use of hormone therapy. Hormone therapy is not appropriate for all women. Women experiencing menopausal symptoms are encouraged to speak with their health-care professional to determine whether hormone therapy might be the right treatment option for them." Despite the dramatic reduction in the number of prescriptions, Wyeth continues to back its HRT medications, implicitly conveying the twenty-first-century pharmaceutical mantra, "Ask your doctor if HRT is right for you."

In a published press release in 2004 regarding the early termination of the estrogen-only trial, the NIH, the sponsor and conductor of the Women's Health Initiative, noted that Wyeth-Ayerst provided the active estrogen for the estrogen-alone study and funded the Women's Health Initiative Memory Study (WHIMS).[45] The pharmaceutical companies have long had a vested interest in research that further supports their products, such as the positive findings from observational studies during the 1980s that led Wyeth to petition the FDA to label estrogen as being "protective against heart disease."[46] The WHI 2002 findings created a major public problem for the drug companies. One month following the July 2002 findings, Bruce Burlington, vice president of regulatory compliance for Wyeth, noted that many of the WHI risks had already been included on the Prempro label and that the study only "better quantified" the risks.[47] Despite their effort to minimize drug risks, Wyeth agreed with the FDA that it was the company's responsibility to "get new information out there" and took actions to convey that information.[48]

Although approximately 5,300 lawsuits from patients claiming HRT caused them serious injury have been filed since the 2002 WHI research was publicized, the first trial did not occur until August 2006. 24 of 31 cases alleging HRT caused breast cancer have been resolved in Wyeth's favor as of March 2009. Of the remaining seven, four cases were settled. One case ruled in favor of three Reno plaintiffs for $35 million in compensatory damages and $99 million in punitive damages, which Wyeth appealed and is awaiting further judgment.[49] The remaining potential 5,000 trials could have a huge impact upon Wyeth's profits since the company is still undergoing lawsuits from Fen-Phen. However, at the current pace, it will be many years before most of the lawsuits are settled. Wyeth has chosen to handle the numerous lawsuits as they are processed by the courts; they have not taken an active role in seeking settlements for them. This further confirms their attempts to maintain a more subtle form of damage control over the situation, possibly hoping that time will diminish some of the negativity of the WHI findings and lead to more settlements in their favor.

The results of the WHI study, the ensuing news reports, and the reaction from the medical community produced a major risk scare for HRT, creating confusion and occasionally panic for some of the estimated 15 million American women taking HRT at the time.[50] As noted earlier, the response to this risk scare was a 43% decline in eighteen months in the number of prescriptions for all oral forms of estrogen — estrogen alone and estrogen/progestin (see figure 5.2).[51]

Within one month of the WHI publication, investigators from the NIH conducted a national random-digit-dialing telephone survey of 819 women. Already, 13% of women had discontinued HRT.[52] In the first six to nine months after the release of the WHI results, 32–56% declines in HRT use were reported by a California health maintenance organization; a California mammography registry; a prescription database study from Ontario, Canada; and a general clinical practice survey from New Zealand. Use of Prempro, the combination estrogen plus progestin studied in the early terminating WHI portion, declined by 80%. Prescriptions for the estrogen-only product Premarin, which was used in the continuing WHI portion of women with a prior hysterectomy, declined by a more modest 48%, presumably due to the continuation of this part of the clinical trial and a perception of less risk for estrogen alone.[53] Other estrogen-containing products demonstrated a smaller 26% decline in prescription rates by the end of 2003. However, despite these dramatic decreases following the WHI results, still over 50% of HRT users — recent estimates range between 4.3 and 10 million women aged 40 to 80 years — continue taking the medication.[54]

Largely due to the pressure of lawsuits, coupled with the responses of the medical profession and the public, overall pharmaceutical company promotional expenditures for standard-dose HRT and ERT preparations have decreased in office detailing, samples, hospitals, and advertising in medical journals since July 2002. However, promotional spending for the "safer" lower-dose preparations of Premarin and

Prempro increased by $20 million during 2003.[55] Preliminary evidence suggests that HRT usage may be increasing with the supposedly "safer" drugs that do not yet have long-term safety data to support this claim. There has been a modest increase in the number of prescriptions of these products, from 0.7 million in July 2002 to 0.9 million at the end of 2003.[56] Another study found that, despite Premarin use dropping by 33% to a monthly prescription rate of 1.8 million in 2002, lower-dose Premarin use increased 6% by the end of 2002.[57] The pharmaceutical companies realize the continued importance of HRT in the medicalization of menopause. They appear to vigorously promote low-dose Prempro and Premarin in response to the most recent HRT risk scare. One set of observers proposed that these marketing trends "suggest a corporate strategy that recognized the importance of the WHI E+P results but also envisioned a continuing and viable market for hormone therapy."[58] And the marketing may be beginning to pay off. Wyeth's yearly earnings report for 2008 showed a 1% gain, or $1,070 million dollars, for the "Premarin Family." It appears that Wyeth is continuing to profit despite the shift in risks for individual women.

MEDICALIZATION, RISK SCARES, AND INDIVIDUALIZED RISK

Over several decades, HRT went from a treatment primarily for symptoms of menopause to a preventive intervention that was meant to reduce the risks of a variety of serious medical disorders. The tragic irony of the 2002 risk scare was the discovery that HRT treatment not only didn't prevent risk, it actually increased the risk of serious diseases and disorders. This led to a steep decrease in the utilization of HRT medications. What impact did this risk scare have on the medicalization of menopause and on the potential and continuance of HRT treatments?

Clearly, doctors reduced their prescribing, and many women stopped taking HRT medications. But roughly half the number of women continued to take their HRT despite the newly identified risks. Medical organizations recommended HRT only for severe menopausal symptoms and only for relatively short periods of time on the lowest possible dose. As with the 1975 HRT risk scare, the response of the pharmaceutical industry has been both defensive and offensive. Defensively, they want to protect themselves against the weight of the oncoming lawsuits, and offensively, they want to maintain their markets by minimizing the associated risks. Thus, as before with the introduction of progesterone in the 1980s, the pharmaceutical companies are looking to produce the "safer" low-dose formulation of HRT so that they can continue to promote their products in the menopause market.

In terms of medicalization, while the risk scare certainly reduced the number of women receiving medical treatments for menopause, it has not substantially affected the definition of menopause. Menopause remains largely medicalized, a "disorder" only awaiting a new and "safer" medication to better treat the symptoms of the condition. If and when such medications are produced, it seems likely, just as in the aftermath of the 1975 HRT risk scare, the prescribing and uptake of HRT will again rise sharply. Pharmaceutical companies, physicians, and consumers, with the sanction of the FDA, would again all contribute to promoting and using this putatively safer drug until new risks to patients are uncovered.

What we see is a pattern of persistent large-scale marketing for HRT that, although periodically reduced by risk scares, is not eliminated by the adverse medical risks of estrogen and progestin. In the current situation, HRT is no longer recommended for all women as a lifetime treatment. But demedicalization would occur only if menopause reverted to a "normal condition," one no longer deemed appropriate for any medical intervention.[59] The continued definition of menopause itself as a medical risk makes women vulnerable to medical interventions and their attendant pharmaceutical risks.

Given the established medical definition of menopause, the pharmaceutical industry has a great incentive to engage in research for menopausal drugs and will continue to tout the known benefits of HRT while awaiting further promising drugs. The medicalized market for menopause treatment is well established, a fact that doesn't escape the pharmaceutical industry. Meanwhile, the FDA maintains its constrained role in evaluating the "safety" of HRT, given its reliance on results from conducted and reported trials with limited access and availability. Thus, the interplay between private (pharmaceutical industry) and public (FDA) interests persists, with the private having significantly greater resources than the public for promoting their positions.

The risks related to HRT have also shifted. Where women took HRT in the 1980s and 1990s to minimize the risk of adverse events, now they have to bear the additional risks of adverse outcomes to treat their menopausal symptoms. While the risk to any individual woman may be low, the population risk is substantial. If the current level of HRT prescription rates were to remain constant, continuing the medicalization of menopause, it is estimated that there would be 6,500 adverse events (heart attacks, strokes, breast cancer, and pulmonary embolisms) attributable to HRT each year.[60] This increase in risk falls on the individual women, abetted by their medical providers, who continue to take HRT despite the changing medical and public views about the efficacy or safety of the treatment.

NOTES

1   Peter Conrad, "Medicalization and Social Control," *Annual Review of Sociology* 18 (1992): 209–32; Peter Conrad, *The Medicalization of Society: On the Transformation of Human Conditions into Medical Disorders* (Baltimore: Johns Hopkins University Press, 2007).

2   Conrad, *Medicalization of Society.*

3   Susan Bell, "Changing Ideas: The Medicalization of Menopause," *Social Science and Medicine* 24, no. 6 (1987): 535–42; Conrad, "Medicalization and Social Control," 209–32; Francis B. McCrea, "The Politics of Menopause: The 'Discovery' of a Deficiency Disease," *Social Problems* 31, no. 1 (1983): 111–23.

4   Bell, "Changing Ideas," 535–42.

5   Michelle P. Warren, "Historical Perspectives in Post-menopausal Hormone Therapy: Defining the Right Dose and Duration," *Mayo Clinic Proceedings* 82, no. 2 (2007): 219–26.

6   Bell, "Changing Ideas," 535–42.

7   Emil Novak, "The Management of the Menopause," *American Journal of Obstetrics and Gynecology* 40 (1940): 594.

8   Catherine Kohler Riessman, "Women and Medicalization: A New Perspective," *Social Policy* 14 (1983): 3–18.

9   Robert A. Wilson, *Feminine Forever* (New York: M. Evans and Company, 1966).

10 McCrea, "Politics of Menopause," 111–23.

11 I. Palmlund, "The Marketing of Estrogens for Menopausal and Postmenopausal Women," *Journal of Psychosomatic Obstetrics and Gynecology* 18 (1997): 158–64.

12 Ibid.

13 McCrea, "Politics of Menopause," 111–23; Adam L. Hersh, Marcia L. Stefanick, and

Randall S. Stafford, "National Use of Postmenopausal Hormone Therapy: Annual Trends and Responses to Recent Evidence," *Journal of the American Medical Association* 291, no. 1 (2004): 47–53.

14 McCrea, "Politics of Menopause," 111–23.

15 Ibid., 115.

16 Ibid., 111–23.

17 Ibid., 116.

18 Amanda Spake, "The Hormone Conundrum," *U.S. News & World Report* 1113, no. 3 (2002).

19 Trisha Gura, "Estrogen: Key Player in Heart Disease Among Women," *Science* 269 (1995): 771–73; Vicki F. Meyer, "The Medicalization of Menopause," *International Journal of Health Services* 31, no. 4 (2001): 769–92.

20 *Harvard Women's Health Watch*, "Postmenopausal Hormones: Where Do We Go From Here?" (newsletter, Harvard Health Publications, January 2003).

21 Palmlund, "Marketing of Estrogens," 158–64.

22 Conrad, *Medicalization of Society*.

23 Anne Katz, "Observations and Advertising: Controversies in the Prescribing of Hormone Replacement Therapy," *Health Care for Women International* 24 (2003): 927–39.

24 Ibid.

25 Meyer, "Medicalization of Menopause," 769–92.

26 Hersh, Stefanick, and Stafford, "National Use," 47–53.

27 Barbara Seaman, *The Greatest Experiment Ever Performed on Women: Exploding the Estrogen Myth* (New York: Hyperion, 2003).

28 Writing Group for the Women's Health Initiative Investigators, "Risks and Benefits of Estrogen Plus Progestin in Healthy Postmenopausal Women: Principal Results from the Women's Health Initiative Randomized Controlled Trial," *Journal of the American Medical Association* 288 (2002): 321–33.

29 Hersh, Stefanick, and Stafford, "National Use," 47–53.

30 Rowan T. Chlebowski et al., "Influence of Estrogen Plus Progestin on Breast Cancer and Mammography in Healthy Postmenopausal Women: The Women's Health Initiative Randomized Trial," *Journal of the American Medical Association* 289 (2003): 3243–53.

31 Jennifer Hays et al., "Effects of Estrogen Plus Progestin on Health-Related Quality of Life," *New England Journal of Medicine* 348, no. 19 (2003): 1839–54.

32 Hersh, Stefanick, and Stafford, "National Use," 47–53.

33 Writing Group for the Women's Health Initiative Investigators, "Effects of

Conjugated Equine Estrogen in Postmenopausal Women with Hysterectomy: The Women's Health Initiative Randomized Controlled Trial," *Journal of the American Medical Association* 291 (2004): 1701–12.

34 Million Women Study Collaborators, "Breast Cancer and Hormone-replacement Therapy in the Million Women Study," *Lancet* 362, no. 9382 (2003): 419–427.

35 Mary C. Brucker and Ellis Quinn Youngkin, "What's a Woman to Do?: Exploring HRT Questions Raised by the Women's Health Initiative," *AWHONN Lifelines* 6, no. 5 (October/November 2002): 408–17.

36 Lisa M. Schwartz and Steven Woloshin, "The Media Matter: A Call for Straightforward Media Reporting," *Annals of Internal Medicine* 140, no. 3 (2004): 226–28.

37 Karen C. Swallen, "Newspaper Coverage of the 1998 Aspirin and 2002 Hormone Therapy Randomized Clinical Trials," Working Paper No. 2003-06 (Center for Demography and Ecology, University of Wisconsin-Madison, 2003).

38 Schwartz and Woloshin, "The Media Matter," 226–28; Hersh, Stefanick, and Stafford, "National Use," 47–53; Sumit R. Majumdar, Elizabeth A. Almasi, and Randall S. Stafford, "Promotion and Prescribing of Hormone Replacement Therapy After Report of Harm by the Women's Health Initiative," *Journal of the American Medical Association* 292, no. 16 (2004): 1983–88.

39 Schwartz and Woloshin, "The Media Matter," 226–28.

40 Jennifer S. Haas et al., "Average Household Exposure to Newspaper Coverage about the Harmful Effects of Hormone Therapy and Population-Based Declines in Hormone Therapy Use," *Journal of General Internal Medicine* 22 (2007): 68–73.

41 FDA, "FDA Statement on the Results of the Women's Health Initiative: Women's Health Initiative (WHI) Results Signal Need for Reassessment of Risks and Benefits of Conjugated Equine Estrogens/medroxyprogesterone Acetate (Prempro) in Postmenopausal Women," (press release, August 12, 2002), http://www.fda.gov/Drugs/DrugSafety/InformationbyDrugClass/ucm135331.htm.

42 The North American Menopause Society, "Estrogen and Progestrogen Use in Peri- and Postmenopausal Women: September 2003 Position Statement of the North American Menopause Society," *Menopause* 10, no. 6 (2003): 497–506; American College of Obstetrics and Gynecologists, "Response to the Women's Health Initiative Study Results," (press release, November 7, 2002), http://www.obgynzisow.com/ACOG%20WHI%20Final%20Report.pdf.

43 Wyeth Pharmaceuticals, "Wyeth Updates Product Labels for its Postmenopausal Hormone Therapies," (press release, September 4, 2002), http://www.wyeth.com/news/archive?nav=display&navTo=/wyeth_html/home/news/pressreleases/2002/1145754912335.html.

44 Ibid.

45 National Institutes of Health, "NIH Asks Participants in Women's Health Initiative Estrogen-Alone Study to Stop Study Pills, Begin Follow-up Phase" (press release, March 2, 2004), http://www.nhlbi.nih.gov/new/press/04-03-02.htm.

46 Ceci Connolly, "Doctors Working to Clear the Fog of Hormone Study," *Washington Post*, July 28, 2002.

47 Marc Kaufman, "Hormone Replacement Gets New Scrutiny: Findings of Increased Risks Prompts Federal Effort," *Washington Post*, August 14, 2002.

48 Ibid.

49 Martha Bellisle, "Federal Judge Moves Lawsuit Against Drug Makers to State Court," *Reno Gazette-Journal*, March 17, 2009.

50 Hersh, Stefanick, and Stafford, "National Use," 47–53.

51 Majumdar, Almasi, and Stafford, "Promotion and Prescribing," 1983–88.

52 Erica S. Breslau et al., "The Hormone Therapy Dilemma: Women Respond," *Journal of the American Medical Women's Association* 58, no. 1 (2003): 33–43.

53 Majumdar, Almasi, and Stafford, "Promotion and Prescribing," 1983–88.

54 Hersh, Stefanick, and Stafford, "National Use," 47–53; Haas et al., "Average Household Exposure," 68–73; Majumdar, Almasi, and Stafford, "Promotion and Prescribing," 1983–88.

55 Majumdar, Almasi, and Stafford, "Promotion and Prescribing," 1983–88.

56 Ibid.

57 Hersh, Stefanick, and Stafford, "National Use," 47–53.

58 Majumdar, Almasi, and Stafford, "Promotion and Prescribing," 1987.

59 Conrad, "Medicalization and Social Control," 225.

60 Jennifer S. Haas et al., "Changes in the Use of Postmenopausal Hormone Therapy after the Publication of Clinical Trial Results," *Annals of Internal Medicine* 140, no. 3 (2004): 184–88.

Toward Safer Prescribing and Better Drugs

DONALD W. LIGHT

Employers, taxpayers, and patients are beginning to realize that the rising costs of prescription drugs stem from higher-priced newer drugs that offer few proven advantages over older, cheaper, similar agents, even as they put patients at greater risk for adverse reactions, as described in Chapter 1. These costs reflect a regulator unable to protect the public adequately, for reasons explained in Chapter 2. Chapter 3 uses the over-prescribing of statins for healthy people to illustrate how physicians are allowing their best clinical judgment to be commercialized. Setting guidelines for "high" cholesterol is one of several examples where expert panels with commercial ties have broadened criteria so that tens of millions more people are designated as "high risk." Revised U.S. guidelines increased the number of people for whom statins are recommended from 13 to 36 million; yet clinical trials not only provided no evidence of a clinical benefit, they showed evidence of serious risk.[1] Company-sponsored studies often lie behind expanding the designation of "high risk" patients, and they are about four times more likely than independent studies to come to conclusions favorable to their funders.[2]

Chapter 4 describes another large area of over-prescribing based on the medicalization of natural responses to life's difficulties. Chapter 5 looks back at the medicalization of menopause and its company-promoted myths. These are just three of many conditions that have been found to be overblown by commercial campaigns, resulting in millions of people swallowing chemicals unnecessarily that bear risks of adverse reactions and cost billions of dollars.[3] They include high blood pressure, attention deficit disorder, social anxiety disorder, and osteoporosis.

What people want from pharmaceutical companies are new drugs that are better than existing ones and that will reduce their pain, control a clinical condition, or cure them—without putting them at serious risk of toxic side effects. There are several ways to reduce consumer risk and reward the development of superior drugs:

1. Reduce exposure to undue risks from existing drugs by reining in the drivers of medicalization.
2. Reduce commercial influences on physicians.
3. Flag and limit prescribing for unapproved uses to situations where there are few alternatives.
4. Empower patients to report side effects as part of a stronger sentinel safety system.
5. Determine the comparative effectiveness of drugs and other interventions.
6. Require that new drugs be better than existing ones as part of a new social contract with companies.
7. Reduce the financial risk that patients now have to bear by fostering competition for value.

We need a stronger, independent Food and Drug Administration (FDA). Public funding for large clinical trials would lower risk and costs for companies and allow prices to be lower. This would create a steadier, profitable business environment less subject to the large losses of failed large trials and the all-out efforts to compensate by generating blockbuster sales from drugs that can result in a crisis of seriously harmed patients, then plummeting sales, and thousands of lawsuits.

DEMEDICALIZE HEALTH PROBLEMS AND EXPOSURE TO RISK

The medicalization of life's emotional stresses as due to biomedical imbalances or of menopause as a "deficiency disease" that calls for hormone replacement therapy (HRT) are just two examples of disease- and fear-mongering that lead millions of people to put themselves at unnecessary risk from swallowing drugs they do not need. As Chapter 5 concludes, the continued ingestion of HRT drugs shown to be dangerous and not therapeutic means that about 6,500 women will experience a heart attack, stroke, breast cancer, or pulmonary embolism each year. Ironically, they trust that their doctors are prescribing in their best interests.

Besides creating diseases where none exist, company-supported advocates have lowered the threshold for treatment for real risks like high blood pressure. Often, patients are not told about studies showing that regular exercise, a Mediterranean diet, less drinking and smoking, and weight control are more effective than prescription drugs.[4] These alternatives also improve alertness, sleep quality, and well-being.

Although cholesterol was hardly mentioned a generation ago as a key risk factor, it is now the dominant concern in preventing heart disease. The pharmaceutical industry and its entourage of researchers, clinical leaders, and writers have promoted concern about high cholesterol along with the taking of statin drugs to the point that they have become the best-selling class of prescription drugs in the United States. Yet a study of 25,000 executives and professional men found that being physically unfit "accounted for three times as many deaths from cardiovascular disease as did elevated cholesterol." Further, "normal-weight men with elevated cholesterol levels had no additional risk [of death from any cause], but the unfit men had a 60 percent higher risk of death."[5] Taking a drug, it would seem, is secondary to exercising. Yet physicians talk to their patients much more often about taking a statin than exercise or smoking cessation. John Abramson, a clinical instructor at Harvard Medical School, concludes, "Doctors and patients are being distracted from what the research really shows: physical fitness, smoking cessation, and a healthy diet trump nearly every medical intervention as the best way to keep coronary heart disease at bay."[6]

The same picture emerges from evidence about type 2 diabetes, a significant cause of kidney failure, stroke, and heart disease. A major study showed that 91% of risk for developing type 2 diabetes was attributed to being overweight, lack of exercise, smoking, and an unhealthy diet. Abramson points out that improving these behavioral causes gets little or no mention by the industry-supported American Diabetes Association and American College of Cardiology. Yet more than two-thirds of diabetics do not get adequate exercise—if they did, their death rate would drop by 39%. Walking two hours or more a week reduces chances of death four times more than taking a statin drug. Losing weight is five times more effective. By contrast, the largest long-term study demonstrated that tight control of blood sugar does not reduce the major macrovascular complications of diabetes.[7]

Obesity is treated more with a variety of costly drugs than by reducing caloric intake, eating more vegetables and fruits, and exercising. Depression and social anxiety get short-term symptomatic relief from drugs, but lasting benefits come from exercise and lifestyle changes. And then there are drugs like Fosamax, Miacalcin, Forteo, or the new class of SERMs (selective estrogen-receptor modulators) that companies heavily promote to reduce "bone loss" and thus reduce broken bones from falls. But bone *mass* naturally declines slowly with age and is a small contributor to the likelihood of broken bones. Exercises for strength and balance to minimize falls and taking calcium and vitamin D are more helpful, as is making high-risk places like the bathroom or kitchen safer.

This summary provides a few examples of over-medicalized problems. *Selling Sickness, The Loss of Sadness, Hooked,* and *The Medicalization of Society* provide other examples.[8] Exposure to the risks of toxic side effects as well as to costly bills could be substantially reduced if we reduced the medicalization of common health problems and the taking of drugs for them. But how do we demedicalize health problems in a world in which two-thirds of patient groups receive funding from drug companies, published studies understate harms and overstate benefits, expert panels who set guidelines are made up of specialists with financial ties to drug companies, and most of the medical societies that run courses and conferences receive large contributions from drug companies?[9]

Concerned citizens and physicians and some congressmen, like Charles Grassley, Max Baucus, John Dingell, and Henry Waxman, are clearly worried. They give examples of companies burying evidence of risks and harms to patients, paying task-force members who endorse a dangerous drug against evidence, and marketing even after they know products are dangerous. As a concerned physician, John Abramson concludes, "The need for drugs will be determined largely by industry-sponsored research, industry-sponsored guidelines, industry-sponsored continuing education and marketing for doctors, and industry-sponsored advertising and public relations campaigns."[10] Worse, more than half the budget of the FDA for reviewing new drug applications comes from company fees, and experts with financial ties are allowed on the FDA advisory committees. Even officials at the National Institutes of Health (NIH) "are allowed to participate in lucrative consulting contracts with the drug companies."[11] The industry has blocked proposals for studies of comparative effectiveness or cost-effectiveness because many of the best-selling drugs may prove little better, but riskier, than cheaper alternatives.

Advertising to patients involves inherently commercialized, biased information. Many physicians as well as independent studies support rules adopted in most countries, and which had existed in the United States for decades, that prohibit or minimize direct marketing to patients. A systematic review of how drug ads affected patients found that less than 1% of the studies cited used randomized or controlled methods and none reported benefits in health outcomes, but the ads did result in more requests for the product and more patients taking it.[12] That is what ads are supposed to do — persuade people through hopes and fears and fantasies to buy more of the product. An analysis of TV ads found that only 26% described risk factors, none mentioned lifestyle changes as an alternative to taking the drug, and more than half portrayed the drug as a breakthrough.[13] Ads concentrate on new products for common chronic conditions, the least likely to be breakthroughs and most likely to shift millions of patients from older drugs to higher-priced new ones, as might be expected. As we saw in Chapter 2, the FDA is incapable of keeping ads from being biased when the point of marketing is to persuade people to do things they would not otherwise do. Medicine should be based on science and independent professional judgment.

The wider need beyond curtailing infomercials is for an independent source of trustworthy information based on non-commercial assessments of evidence about dangers and benefits of treatment options. This leads some physicians to recommend a publicly funded Institute of Medical Science. Others propose a center for the study of comparative effectiveness or an institute for clinical trials, but the Institute of Medical Science idea addresses the wider scope of commercialized, medicalized knowledge at all levels, from a physician addressing the needs of a patient to the creation of unbiased knowledge in world-class journals. This view is supported by the new report on conflict of interest from the

Institute of Medicine, which finds conflict of interest at every level of health care, from medical students to deans to the National Institutes of Health, and recommends that it be eliminated.[14]

An Institute of Medical Science could be modeled on the Federal Reserve Board to maximize insulation from political and commercial influence—secure funding from Congress, no financial ties to industry, and long, staggered terms. It could be a source of authoritative knowledge for health professionals, the press, and the public. It would provide oversight in developing guidelines for prevention, diagnosis, and treatment through independent analyses of all scientific evidence. It would foster transparency and require that medical research be designed, conducted, and analyzed according to scientific standards and directed at improving health. It would fund and oversee research on issues where good evidence is lacking. And it could assess the comparative effectiveness and cost-effectiveness of new therapies to minimize the privatization of clinical and financial risks.

REDUCE COMMERCIAL INFLUENCE ON PHYSICIANS

Drug companies spend billions of dollars on physicians to persuade them to depart from their own clinical judgment in prescribing; this commercial influence is so great that it can overcome solid evidence that a drug is dangerous. For example, the New York Times published an article about the paltry impact of a six-year independent study completed in 2002 of newer and older drugs for hypertension, the ALLHAT (Antihypertensive and Lipid-Lowering Treatment to Prevent Heart Attack Trial) study. It found that Norvasc (a Pfizer drug) increased chances of heart failure by 38% with few offsetting benefits compared to old diuretics that cost one-twentieth as much.[15] AstraZeneca's ACE inhibitor was also more risky, and Pfizer's Cardura doubled the risk of hospitalization for health failure. Like company responses to evidence that Vioxx was dangerous (see Chapter 1) and to evidence that HRT did more harm than good (see Chapter 5), Pfizer issued scripted responses for sales reps to reassure doctors that Cardura was safe and to downplay or recast ALLHAT's negative findings. In a medical ad it turned the negative findings of the authoritative study on their head by proclaiming "ALL HATs off" to its drug. Pfizer's CEO said, "Allhat is extremely positive for Norvasc." Spin trumped science and safety. Sales *increased*, from $3.7 billion in 2002 (when the study results were published) to $4.9 billion in 2006. Based on the trial results, this means that many more patients were exposed to serious risks of heart failure by taking expensive drugs that provided no advantage over diuretics.[16]

We saw the same ability to sell dangerous drugs in Chapter 5 with HRT and with Vioxx in Chapter 1. Henry Waxman's report on the marketing materials that Congress required Merck to submit describes how the company neutralized evidence of cardiovascular risk associated with Vioxx published on the front page of the *New York Times* and on the FDA Web site by simply asserting the opposite. Physicians apparently believed Merck sales reps more than the *New York Times* and wrote even more prescriptions. We see this same dynamic today. In July 2009, the FDA approved Multaq for treating a heart rhythm disorder that affects 7 million people in the United States and Europe. According to the *New York Times*, despite its being less effective than an existing drug, amiodarone, and having a fivefold increase in the risk of stroke and a black box warning, Sanofi-Aventis anticipates it will be able to get physicians to prescribe $2 billion of Multaq a year.[17] They are masters of marketing and are probably right. Is the lesson that heavy marketing puts patients at risk and should be limited?

The medical profession has grown concerned about the loss of public trust and the commercialization of professional practice. It has organized efforts to restore professionalism and patient trust, such as White Coat ceremonies for medical students to dedicate themselves to healing patients and stronger standards about accepting gifts, trips, and other favors.[18] As many distinguished physicians have emphasized, including Howard Brody in this volume, these efforts do not seem to come close to what is needed to restore independent clinical judgment. A number of major medical centers and schools are limiting or prohibiting access by sales reps to medical students, residents, and faculty because they have come to realize reps undermine their credibility as leaders in scientific medicine and can distort medical education. For example, Massachusetts General Hospital and affiliates of Partners Healthcare implemented stricter rules in 2009 that will direct all free samples to general repositories and prohibit their doctors from joining industry speakers' bureaus, an easy source of generous fees for giving talks to colleagues designed to increase prescribing a new drug.[19]

The lone maverick initiative, No Free Lunch, started by Columbia University internist Jeff Goodman, has evolved into a national movement. Physicians can take the No Free Lunch Pledge and get listed as "promotion-free." Under a "pen amnesty" program, they can send in their pens with the names of drugs or companies and get back a pen with the No Free Lunch logo. The No Free Lunch Web site offers excellent information and a network of other physicians who believe that all gifts large and small compromise the fiduciary relationship with their patients. The public can look up "promotion-free doctors." Concerned medical students at the American Medical Student Association pull no punches scoring how commercialized their instructors and schools have become. Only nine of the 149 medical schools scored received an A; thirty-five received a C or D, including Duke and Tufts; and another thirty-five received an F, including Tulane.[20]

PharmedOut.org is a newer and more extensive organization that was created with a $21 million grant from a lawsuit settlement between state attorneys general and Warner-Lambert, a division of Pfizer, for its off-label promotion of Neurontin (gabapentin). It offers commercial-free continuing medical education courses and a No Drug Rep Certificate that a practice can display, letting patients know it "does not allow visits from pharmaceutical salespeople because we rely on scientific information, not marketing, to decide what treatment is best for you."

In addition, several states have passed laws mandating that companies make public their payments to physicians.[21] Although they reflect an unprecedented level of concern, companies are circumventing these initiatives. Some companies have undermined the effort by claiming payments to physicians are trade secrets.[22] Even when reported, the name of the recipient is not usually included, and in some states the information is not made public. Some companies are doing their own disclosure by setting up online databases of payments to doctors.

Two states, Pennsylvania and Maine, have gone further and established state-funded academic detailing, that is, reps who counter the influence of company reps by visiting physicians to talk about the latest new drugs but based on independent evidence of their efficacy and risks. The Senate Committee on Aging has written a bill to create academic detailing on a national level, as is done in some other countries.[23]

Responding to public discontent and congressional hearings, many pharmaceutical companies have also volunteered to cut back on gifts to physicians. Even small gifts set up the psychological association of the brand drug with the gift and the obligation implicit in a gift-relationship to reciprocate by prescribing it.[24] The industry's trade association has updated its voluntary code of conduct, limiting the size of gifts, meals, trips, and other favors, and it has separated grant-giving from marketing.[25] Many companies have signed the code. If effective, this could address the heart of the risk proliferation syndrome described in Chapter 1, in which companies fund a range of market-driven studies and trials as a way to recruit leading clinicians, pay them well, and position them to be the sponsored speakers at courses, conferences, and grand rounds to promote expanded concepts of health problems and prescribing that expose more patients to the risks of prescription drugs.

These unprecedented pledges to decommercialize physician prescribing include pharmaceutical companies separating grants for continuing medical education from marketing departments. Although companies are doing this, the Senate Committee on Finance reported that pharmaceutical companies use "educational grants to help build market share for their newer and more lucrative products." This drives up costs and puts patients at risk because new products "have less clinical history and may expose patients to greater risks than older products with better established safety and efficacy."[26] Of particular concern are unapproved or off-label uses that companies cannot promote directly but can promote through third-party intermediaries over whom the FDA has no jurisdiction. In response, the Senate Committee undertook months of investigation.

The committee found that "a multi-billion dollar industry of for-profit medical education and communication companies has developed to run medical education programs sponsored by drug companies."[27] The organizational separation of marketing from professional education is based on the premise that companies will pay for physicians' continuing education without influencing the content. But why should they? In fact, the committee reports that marketing departments serve as gatekeepers and selectors, and the "independent" medical education companies know what to do to win future contracts. While the new rules and reforms no longer allow marketing departments to provide these grants, they determine which proposals are of interest to "ensure that the Company's grant making is consistent with its business strategy."[28] "The information presented often encourages physicians to change their prescribing practices to favor certain drugs," the committee reports; yet this is what the ostensible separation of marketing from educational grants is supposed to prevent.[29]

Commercialized information becomes *more* influential, in fact, because it gains "an imprimatur of credibility and independence" by being delivered in the context of "education." Likewise, while the anti-kickback law prohibits companies from paying doctors to prescribe their products for patients with Medicare or Medicaid, the committee reports that *de facto* kickbacks through the medical education companies are allowed and occur "where companies overpay high-prescribing physicians as 'consultants' or 'speakers' for minimal work to develop educational material or teach at educational programs."[30] The accreditation process for courses and providers leaves room for commercial influence because 80% compliance with criteria is deemed satisfactory. Educational grants are also used to fund the development of clinical guidelines, which have been instrumental in expanding the number of patients taking drugs and being exposed to their risks. Thus professional education remains deeply commercialized and a principal means for promoting unapproved uses.

Few other professions have company-sponsored courses, and they are entirely unnecessary. Lawyers, accountants, sociologists, and even nurses pay for courses to update or improve their knowledge. As Marcia Angell, the past editor-in-chief of the *New England Journal of Medicine*, puts it, "Get Big Pharma Out of Medical Education."[31]

LIMIT PRESCRIBING FOR UNAPPROVED USES

Because about three-quarters of off-label uses are not supported by good evidence of their effectiveness, they put patients at risk for adverse reactions without offsetting benefits. They also undermine the regulatory system that tries to minimize the privatization of risk by testing drugs for safety and effectiveness. Thus the problem is not just the off-label uses but their systemic effect on the whole public enterprise to protect the public from privatized risks. Once new drugs are well-established through the commercialized education syndrome of courses, professional meetings, and personal visits by reps, companies are inclined to exploit the blurred line between clinical trials for approval and other less rigorous trials to provide evidence for unapproved uses and market indirectly from there. If doctors, who can prescribe any drug for any use, get most of their information about drugs from commercial sources promoting them, and if companies promote to the widest range of physicians to maximize sales, such as promoting psychotropic drugs to general internists and family physicians as well as psychiatrists, it makes one wonder what role is left for the FDA to play in protecting patients from avoidable risks without benefits. The myth is that the companies test for the main effect of a drug and are prohibited from marketing it for anything else. The reality is that companies test for an endpoint that will get a drug approved and then market it for other indications through paid intermediaries, especially clinical leaders, so that they do not violate the letter of the law.

Supporting this syndrome is the lack of testing for whole sub-populations, especially children, so that off-label uses become unavoidably routine. After drug companies refused for years to test drugs for children, Congress granted a six-month extension of exclusive marketing rights for doing so. Companies have responded largely by testing their most profitable drugs, even when they are not very relevant to children, in order to make additional profits and stave off generics from initiating normal price competition. As Dr. Angell writes, "That law is a virtual bribery, and it doesn't even accomplish its stated purpose."[32]

Two other areas where physicians prescribe for unauthorized uses are for patients with chronic conditions who are constantly looking for something better than what they are taking and patients with life-threatening conditions, like cancer, who want to try anything that any board-certified specialist thinks might work. In both cases, the placebo effect of hope and faith in a recommendation from one's doctor must be powerful. Patients cannot tell and do not want to know that many new cancer drugs offer little additional clinical benefit, though they are heavily promoted among oncologists and patients desperate for a ray of hope and willing to pay thousands for it.[33]

There could be several ways to limit unauthorized uses. One would be to require that physicians and pharmacists tell patients an unapproved use is being recommended and have them sign a statement acknowledging it. Often, physicians do not talk about their recommendation being unapproved or about the pros and cons of the patient taking the drug. An informed consent statement would prompt an explicit occasion for discussing why one's physician is recommending a drug for an unapproved use. Another idea is to have physician drug-reviewing committees in group practices, clinics, and hospitals pass on off-label uses before anyone in the group can prescribe them. This area would benefit from further deliberation and recommendations by the Institute of Medicine.

However, for the first time, new FDA guidelines permit drug companies to distribute to physicians articles about unproven, off-label uses. As Aaron Kesselheim, a prominent physician at Harvard, put it, "If a drug company can go directly to the physician with its published trials without having to go through the FDA first, why would it ever go before the FDA?"[34] Congressman Henry Waxman wrote that the guidelines were "ill-advised" and allow companies to short-circuit FDA review "by sponsoring drug trials that are carefully constructed to deliver positive results and then using the result to influence prescribing patterns."[35] His concern is supported by internal documentation of how Warner-Lambert (now Pfizer) promoted off-label uses of Neurontin by not publishing negative results and having the marketing department orchestrate the publication of positive trials through ghostwritten articles.[36] Two leading experts warn that "there are major limitations in relying on sponsor-distributed literature to regulate off-label use, including the selective publication of studies, the systematic manipulation of the literature, the absence from the literature of critical data necessary for evaluating off-label use, and the potential for undermining the NDA [new drug application] review process."[37] The public and Congress need to limit unapproved uses and keep the FDA from undermining its mandate to protect patients from ineffective and unsafe drugs.

EMPOWER PATIENTS TO REPORT SIDE EFFECTS

In Chapter 2 we summarized the major changes put through by Congress and also within the FDA to strengthen postmarket surveillance. The FDA now has greater authority to require postmarket studies of suspected safety risks, make label changes to add warnings or limit uses, and levy substantial fines. The linking of large data sets and their use to identify patterns of adverse reactions that neither patients nor physicians can discern at the individual level is a promising development. Leading clinicians have called for an independent safety division that has full public funding. The FDA in some ways is taking action to better protect patients from safety risks. For example, in July 2009 it banned two of the most popular prescription painkillers in the world because of liver damage caused by acetaminophen, an ingredient also found in Tylenol and Excedrin.[38] The next day, Johnson and Johnson took out a full-page ad asserting that the drug was perfectly safe if used properly, deflecting attention from the FDA evidence of the drug's toxic effects to the misuse of it.

While the FDA and the companies duke it out, why not empower patients to report side effects directly? Of course, patients do this now in a haphazard way, but most do not know whom to call or e-mail. As a result, over 90% of all adverse reactions do not get reported. Telling their doctor takes time and money—and apparently does not work. We saw in Chapter 1 that patients report adverse effects of drugs that are supported by scientific evidence, and yet their physicians dismiss them. In another study, investigators surveyed hospitalized patients and found that 23% reported at least one significant adverse reaction; yet physicians and nurses reported fewer than half of them in the patient records, even though most were considered clinically significant.[39]

Most of the estimated 46 million adverse reactions (see pp. 2–6) go unreported and are medically minor, but they seriously affect people's ability to work or take care of others or themselves. For example, adverse reactions of a newly approved drug could include diarrhea, nausea, fatigue, and loss of strength. None of these compromises an organ system or is medically serious, but they certainly compromise people's lives. It would not be rocket science to design and field-test a short form for patient feedback. In fact, the Dutch have already developed and tested systemically a simple reporting form that results in patient reports as accurate as reports from professionals.[40] A lack of funds for roll-out has kept this short form from being used widely as a national sentinel system, but it seems worth trying to complement other clinician-based sources and to identify more of the 95–99% of adverse reactions not now reported. A patient reporting form could be put on the Web site home pages of the FDA, the AMA and other medical societies, every pharmaceutical company, and patient organizations. A toll-free number could be posted at checkout counters, retirement homes, restaurants, and educational institutions.

DETERMINE THE COMPARATIVE EFFECTIVENESS OF DRUGS AND OTHER INTERVENTIONS

Comparing the quality of products is natural; we do it all the time in our personal lives. *Consumer Reports* has pioneered its Best Buy Drugs project to bring patients independent comparative assessments of drugs for major health problems based on existing evidence.[41] Its Web site provides a wealth of user-friendly information about drugs based on a national, authoritative analysis. Well-managed health care systems, such as Kaiser and the Veterans Health Administration, also have research departments that compare the effectiveness of different drugs or clinical interventions, but there is limited comparative effectiveness research nationally.

As the performance of the American health care system has declined compared to other advanced countries despite spending much more, pressure has grown to establish a comparative effectiveness research institute. In 2008, senators Max Baucus and Kent Conrad introduced a bill to establish such an institute that would be private, nonprofit, and publicly funded. It would conduct head-to-head studies, largely on drugs. Its larger purpose would be to become a trusted source of reliable information about safety and efficacy. This agenda moved forward rapidly when President Obama signed into law $1.1 billion for comparative effectiveness research (CER) as part of his economic stimulus package in February 2009.

The pharmaceutical and medical device industry and its advocates responded by mounting an intense campaign against it. Apparently companies want to say their new products are "better" without evidence. According to Jerry Avorn, a professor of medicine at Harvard, "The problem is that comparative studies will be threatening to makers and sellers of costly goods and services that offer no benefit over existing alternatives."[42] Opponents raise a number of objections. The deputy commissioner of the FDA reflected industry interests by claiming that the conclusions will be flawed and yet used to restrict payment by Medicare and insurers. However, nothing in the legislation provides for payment restrictions, and no one can know whether CER findings will be flawed before they are undertaken. Would doing no comparative research be therefore less flawed? Congressman Tom Price claims the CER legislation would create "a permanent government rationing board." This is an odd way to characterize preferring safer, more effective procedures. Similar objections are that CER would lead to "cookbook medicine" and to the government forcing physicians to do what it decides is best.[43]

However, good comparative research will not necessarily or even usually mean that patients will be protected from more dangerous drugs because company promotions are so effective at overriding evidence of serious risks. One implication is that patients, consumers, and practitioners should be involved in the design of comparative research and the dissemination of its findings.[44] CER also needs to avoid past mistakes, such as the biased designs, analyses, and presentations of past trials.[45] Research should assess actual clinical effectiveness, not proof of efficacy on surrogate endpoints. Studies should recognize that synthetic chemicals are dangerous and thus measure all adverse reactions, including those that make subjects drop out of a trial, such as organ toxicity. CER will only be as good as the science and clinical relevance of its studies. Finally, CER needs to be accompanied by a stronger insistence that all information to physicians and patients reflect the best objective evidence of clinical benefits and harms.

The lack of incentives for physicians to prescribe cheaper, comparable, or safer drugs also needs to be addressed. More effective than tiered co-payments, which make patients pay more if their doctor prescribes a more costly drug, would be tiered bonus payments to physicians — nothing if they prescribe a drug from the most costly tier within a therapeutic class, $40 if they prescribe from the second tier, and $80 if they prescribe from the cheapest tier.

The English already have NICE, the National Institute for Clinical Evidence, which uses public funding to bring together top research teams to assess the relative effectiveness and cost-effectiveness of new drugs and devices. Their methods and findings are transparent and widely respected, though sometimes controversial when they conclude that a new, very expensive cancer drug is not worth the cost. These decisions are commonly characterized as rationing to deny desperate patients valuable drugs, but this ignores the evidence that the drugs offer little additional benefit at a very high price. What companies charge, or the "cost" of cancer drugs, is the issue, and it puts patients at serious financial risk. For example, we cited systematic evidence that a new generation of cancer drugs offer almost no advantages and yet are priced much higher. American insurers and health plans apparently pay what companies charge, thus rewarding them to develop new drugs with few benefits. We also know that most of the cost and risk of developing cancer drugs is paid by government programs like the NIH, foundations, and other outside sources, leaving companies with unusually low risk and fixed costs. The NIH and others even fund a substantial number of cancer trials, and the trials are both smaller and shorter than for most other drugs.[46] As far as one can tell, the price of cancer drugs should therefore be lower than the price for hay fever drugs, if based on net corporate outlays. Manufacturing costs appear to be somewhat higher, so perhaps a reasonable price might be $10 a dose but not $100 or $1,000 a dose. Companies have provided no basis, aside from rhetoric, for charging so much, but "the market" pays up. One also finds no discussion in the United States of the much lower prices that the same companies charge for the same drugs in other countries that take value pricing seriously, like England, New Zealand, Germany, and Australia. So long as we richly reward companies for new drugs that are little or no better, we will get more of them and put more patients at risk with few offsetting benefits.

In addition to NICE, the English have set aside about $1 billion from their health care budget to conduct comparative trials to answer important clinical questions about how best to use different drugs that companies have no interest in funding, like comparing new brand-name drugs to generic alternatives. The trials will be conducted on a noncommercial basis and run by independent clinical epidemiologists using only randomized designs and hard clinical endpoints. All adverse drug reactions will be recorded and analyzed in order to obtain the fullest possible safety profile. Congress and the Agency for Healthcare Research and Quality could undertake a similar initiative to make prescribing safer and less costly.

REWARD COMPANIES FOR DEVELOPING SAFER, MORE EFFECTIVE DRUGS

Just as it is easier and more profitable for companies to claim their new drugs are therapeutically superior without objective evidence that they are, so current incentives reward companies for developing variations on existing drugs that are little or no better and may expose patients to greater risks. The most obvious problem is that we do not set the benchmark for approving new drugs as better than existing ones but only as better than an inert substance or placebo. Companies respond by giving us what we ask for—lots of new drugs that meet this low standard but little or no better than previous ones did. If we want new drugs to be therapeutically superior, we need to change the criterion for approval and thus the purpose of R&D (research and development)—to develop drugs that add real value for patients.[47] This would greatly reduce patient exposure to side effects, first by guaranteeing genuine clinical advantages to offset risks and second by greatly reducing the number of new drugs that patients take. Marcia Angell makes the important point that not testing against the best effective treatment is unethical.[48]

Requiring that new drugs be better than existing ones means specifying which uses are safer or more effective rather than just approving them. For example, in the case of Vioxx, benefits might have exceeded harms for a small percentage of patients, and the same point now applies to Multaq for atrial fibrillation. But the right of physicians to prescribe a drug for anything is an open invitation for companies to persuade them to prescribe it for conditions where the risks of harm exceed the chances of benefitting.

We also do not get safer, better drugs because even large payers like employers, insurance companies, and Medicare pay much more for new variations, as we saw in the ALLHAT example. If Ford were to come out with a hybrid that was 5% more efficient and charged twice as much for it, no one would buy it, especially commercial buyers who purchase cars by the fleet. But large American insurers pay much more for new drugs that are little or no better than existing ones. For example, the acid reflux drug Nexium is derived from Prilosec, yet Oregon Health and Science University found there is no clinical difference between the two in reducing heartburn. However, insurers cover Nexium at $193 a month without price negotiation, even though Prilosec costs only $19–$26 a month.[49] The common explanation is that drug companies have a patent on a unique product and so they have buyers over a barrel; but this is not true of drugs in the same class. Companies making cars, computers, and cell phones also have patents on their latest innovations and yet compete on value. By contrast, Medicare has expanded payments for cancer drugs used for unapproved indications.[50] This rewards the risk proliferation syndrome and commercialized science. Large buyers and physicians who do not insist on good value reward pharmaceutical companies for developing mostly new drugs of little value. Value purchasing, which is the principal driver of innovation to gain market share by developing something better than the competition, seems absent.

Paying for value and approving only clinically superior drugs would increase companies' already high risks further and reduce their windfall profits from high prices for drugs of little value. Thus, we need to help companies out by offering to pay for clinical trials from public funds. This would further reduce the privatization of risk because all the biased design features of commercial trials listed in Chapter 1 would be eliminated and all adverse reactions would be documented. Transparency and scientific integrity would improve.[51] Already, 84% of all funds for basic research to discover new drugs come from public sources, a figure never cited in the American literature.[52] In addition, the NIH also funds thousands of clinical trials. Merrill Goozner has assembled detailed evidence that much of the risk and cost of drug innovation is borne by public and nonprofit sources.[53] Nevertheless, a revised social contract between the pharmaceutical industry and society would reduce the risks and costs of developing clinically superior and safer drugs so that companies could enjoy steady profits and less boom/bust fluctuation at lower prices. It also would save the industry from itself by forcing it to focus on serious innovation and meeting societal needs.

Nearly every author who has reviewed the current drug approval process calls for an independent institute for drug trials with independent funding. We agree and put the case in terms of a "Better Deal" for drug companies, or a revised social contract. Funding could come from a surcharge of one dollar per prescription. For example, in 2007 there were 3.8 billion prescriptions, so a $1.00 surcharge would yield $3.8 billion for trials.[54] One could either add a $1.00 surcharge to the average price of $69.91 or subtract $1.00 from the $54.53 the manufacturers receive to fund testing of how safe and effective drugs are.

Since manufacturing most pills costs "pennies" as the Congressional Budget Office reported,[55] drug companies would still make large profits. For example, if we assume that most pills cost ten cents to make in volume, then using the 2007 figures, drug companies would gross $203.4 billion ($53.53 x 3.8 billion scripts) minus $0.38 billion in manufacturing costs ($0.10 x 3.8) for a gross profit on cost of goods of $203.0 billion. It is this huge profit that enables companies to spend so much on physicians to get them to prescribe more and so much on the risk proliferation syndrome to expand the "need" for more drugs. It also allows for executive compensation packages, administrative overhead, set-asides for adverse drug reactions, lawsuits, and their portion of R&D.[56] Industry data indicate that companies earn back all R&D and other costs at European prices, plus good profits.[57] In fact, the U.K. government pays drug companies their costs, plus a guaranteed good profit, just from U.K. sales. Sales to the United States, Europe, Japan, and elsewhere are extra. Suppose, for example, that the average prescription price were dropped from $69.91 to $40. Then 3.8 billion prescriptions would yield $152.0 billion and a gross profit on cost of goods of $151.6 billion. This would save Medicare Part D, patients, and anyone else paying for prescriptions $52.4 billion. Using a different, more complex approach, an important study concluded that if all pharmaceutical R&D were federally funded and intellectual property were put in the public domain, the government would more than save the cost in its purchases of drugs.[58]

To carry out reforms to make new drugs more effective and safe, the FDA must be fully funded by Congress and not funded at all by the companies it regulates. To regulate one of the best-paid industries in the world to protect people from hidden risks, salaries for staff must be high and attractive terms established, such as free child care and generous pensions. Promotions need to be based on merit. Other sources of commercial influence need to be minimized, such as prohibitions and penalties against revolving-door careers.

REDUCE FINANCIAL RISK FOR PATIENTS

A reduction in financial risks to patients would follow from reforms that result in fewer patients taking fewer drugs at lower prices and incurring fewer costs from adverse reactions. There is considerable pressure in

STRATEGIES TO MAXIMIZE SALES & PROFITS	STRATEGIES TO MAXIMIZE DRUG SAFETY & EFFECTIVENESS
—Medicalize worries, perceived risks, and "diseases" for which people will take drugs.	—Demedicalize normal risks, variations, and responses to life and emphasize good coping skills and healthy habits.
—Quickly approve as many apparently safe new drugs as possible, whether clinically superior or not, based on trials designed by companies to minimize evidence of harms and maximize evidence of benefits.	—Approve only new drugs proven clinically superior and tested for safety in independent trials designed to detect all adverse events and to identify the lowest effective dosages.
—Use surrogate endpoints around which whole models of risk can be constructed to create new markets of need.	—Use clinical endpoints around health conditions and risks relevant to patients.
—Commercialize professional judgment. Have sales reps be the principal source of information, education, and advice about prescribing. Have marketing departments fund educational courses and professional conference sessions.	—Keep professional judgment independent and scientific. Provide independent educational and advisory materials and help physicians to exercise their best professional judgment of what is best for patients.
—Reward *de facto* proliferation of unapproved uses to maximize sales, fueled by DTCA (direct-to-consumer advertising) and paid physician educators. Mass market for all plausible uses.	—Limit prescribing to approved uses, with provisions for other uses when reviewed by the patient and medical professionals.
—Monitor adverse events primarily through passive, voluntary reporting by the companies that profit from selling the drugs.	—Monitor uses in systematic ways. Analyze data from large clinical data sets for benefits and harms.
—Have an underfunded, understaffed safety division with few powers to investigate and withdraw problem drugs and to warn and protect the public.	—Have a well-funded and well-staffed safety division with independent powers to investigate and withdraw problem drugs and to warn and protect the public.
—Have experts with industry ties set prescribing guidelines that maximize the number of patient-consumers.	—Use independent experts to set guidelines that minimize the number of patients exposed to risks.

Table 6.1   Which model shall prevail?

Washington to remove the prohibition against the government negotiating for lower prices for Medicare patients. If removed, the money saved would allow the Medicare coverage ravine to be filled, as explained in Chapter 1. Marcia Angell flags another source of high costs to patients and payers, a rule that now allows patent-holding companies to file additional patents and then sue generic companies for infringement, which then "triggers successive thirty-month stays on generic competition."[59] The FDA now fully participates by ignoring the legal restriction of such lawsuits to patents listed in the FDA Orange Book. Several other techniques used by patent-holding companies to block or delay normal price competition have been documented in a major report on anti-competitive behavior by the European Commission on Competition.[60] They attest to the companies' legal innovations and dedication to maximizing monopoly protection of company-controlled pricing.

In conclusion, recent initiatives and the proposals here can reduce the 2.3 million hospitalizations and 111,000 deaths from drugs that doctors prescribe that too often have more risks and fewer advantages than people realize. This man-made epidemic calls for serious action. Table 6.1 contrasts the current strategies to maximize sales and profits with strategies to maximize drug safety and effectiveness. Some current changes strengthen safety regulations but do not require that new drugs be more effective (or reward companies for making them so). In fact, some changes have weakened the FDA's ability to be sure new drugs help patients more than they harm them. Isn't it time to change the rules?

NOTES

1   J. Abramson and J. M. Wright, "Are Lipid-Lowering Guidelines Evidence-Based?" *Lancet* 369 (2007): 168–69.

2   Joel Lexchin et al., "Pharmaceutical Industry Sponsorship and Research Outcome and Quality: Systematic Review," *British Medical Journal* 326 (2003): 1167–70.

3   Ray Moynihan and Alan Cassels, *Selling Sickness: How the World's Biggest Pharmaceutical Companies Are Turning Us All into Patients* (New York: Nation Books, 2005).

4   John Abramson, *Overdosed America* (New York: HarperCollins, 2004). The text is based on Chapter 13.

5   Abramson, *Overdosed America*, 222.

6   Abramson, *Overdosed America*, 222.

7 James McCormack and Tricia Greenhalgh, "Seeing What You Want to See in Randomized Controlled Trials: Versions and Perversions of UKPDS Data," *British Medical Journal* 320 (2000): 1720–23; Stephen Havas, "The ACCORD Trial and Control of Blood Glucose Level in Type 2 Diabetes Mellitus: Time to Challenge Conventional Wisdom," *Archives of Internal Medicine* 169, no. 2 (2009): 150–54.

8 Moynihan and Cassels, *Selling Sickness*; Allan V. Horwitz and Jerome C. Wakefield, *The Loss of Sadness* (New York: Oxford University Press, 2007); Howard Brody, *Hooked: Ethics, the Medical Profession, and the Pharmaceutical Industry* (Lanham, MD: Rowman and Littlefield, 2007); Peter Conrad, *The Medicalization of Society: On the Transformation of Human Conditions into Medical Disorders* (Baltimore: Johns Hopkins University Press, 2007).

9 See Chapter 1.

10 Abramson, *Overdosed America*, 245.

11 Abramson, *Overdosed America*, 249.

12 S. Gilbody et al., "Benefits and Harms of Direct to Consumer Advertising: A Systematic Review," *Quality and Safety in Health Care* 14 (2005): 246–50.

13 Dominick L. Frosch et al., "Creating Demand for Prescription Drugs: A Content Analysis of Television Direct-to-Consumer Advertising," *Annals of Family Medicine* 5 (2007): 6–13.

14 Institute of Medicine, *Conflict of Interest in Medical Research, Education, and Practice* (Washington, DC: National Academies Press, 2009).

15 Maggie Mahar and Niko Karvounis, "We Have Comparative Effectiveness Research—Now It's Time to Use It," Health Beat blog, January 20, 2009, http://www.healthbeatblog.org/2008/12/-we-have-comparative-effectiveness-research-now-its-time-to-use-it-.html.

16 Grace E. Jackson, "Open Letter to the Federal Coordinating Council for Comparative Effectiveness Research," Bonkers Institute, April 12, 2009, http://www.bonkersinstitute.org/jacksonletter.html.

17 Duff Wilson, "Sanofi Drug for Heart Rhythm Disorder Is Approved," *New York Times*, July 3, 2009.

18 Troyen Brennan et al., "Health Industry Practices That Create Conflicts of Interest: A Policy Proposal for Academic Medical Centers," *Journal of the American Medical Association* 295 (2006): 429–33; Donald W. Light, "Health Care Professions, Markets, and Countervailing Powers," in *Handbook of Medical Sociology*, 6th edition, ed. Chloe E. Bird et al. (Upper Saddle River, NJ: Prentice Hall, forthcoming), chap. 14.

19 *Boston Globe*, "Pills Without Shills," *Boston Globe*, April 17, 2009, http://www.boston.

com/bostonglobe/editorial_opinion/editorials/articles/2009/04/17/pills_without_shills/.

20 See www.nofreelunch.org and the American Medical Student Association's "AMSA PharmFree Scorecard 2008" at http://amsascorecard.org/.

21 Robert Steinbrook, "Disclosure of Industry Payments to Physicians," *New England Journal of Medicine* 359 (2008): 559–61.

22 Based on Joseph S. Ross et al., "Pharmaceutical Company Payments to Physicians," *Journal of the American Medical Association* 297 (2007): 1216–23.

23 *Independent Drug Education and Outreach Act of 2008*, 110th Cong., 2d sess. (July 31, 2008): S 3396. See http://www.rxfacts.org/pdf/Independent%20Drug%20Education%20Act%20(IDEA).pdf.

24 Dana Katz, Arthur L. Caplan, and Jon Merz, "All Gifts Large and Small: Toward an Understanding of the Ethics of Pharmaceutical Industry Gift Giving," *American Journal of Bioethics* 3, no. 3 (2003): 39–46.

25 PhRMA, *Code on Interactions with Healthcare Professionals* (Washington, DC: Pharmaceutical Research and Manufacturers of America, 2008), http://www.phrma.org/code_on_interactions_with_healthcare_professionals/. See also Mark Gould, "End of the free lunch?" *British Medical Journal* 337 (2008): 487–88.

26 Senate Committee on Finance, *Use of Educational Grants by Pharmaceutical Manufacturers*, 110th Cong., 1st sess., 2007, S. Prt. 110-21, 1.

27 Ibid., 18.

28 Ibid., 11.

29 Ibid., 12.

30 Ibid., 17.

31 Marcia Angell, *The Truth About the Drug Companies: How They Deceive Us and What to Do About It* (New York: Random House, 2004), 250.

32 Ibid., 248.

33 See for example Silvio Garattini and Vittorio Bertele, "Efficacy, Safety, and Cost of New Anticancer Drugs," *British Medical Journal* 325 (2002): 269–71.

34 Mike Mitka, "Critics Say FDA's Off-Label Guidance Allows Marketing Disguised as Science," *Journal of the American Medical Association* 299 (2008): 1759–61.

35 Ibid., 1760.

36 Michael A. Steinman et al., "Narrative Review: The Promotion of Gabapentin: An Analysis of Internal Industry Documents," *Annals of Internal Medicine* 145 (2006): 284–93.

37 Bruce M. Psaty and Wayne Ray, "FDA Guidance on Off-Label Promotion and the State of the Literature From Sponsors," *Journal of the American Medical Association* 299 (2008): 1949.

38 Gardiner Harris, "Ban Is Advised on 2 Top Pills for Pain Relief," *New York Times*, July 1, 2009.

39 Joel S. Weissman et al., "Comparing Patient-Reported Hospital Adverse Events with Medical Record Review: Do Patients Know Something That Hospitals Do Not?" *Annals of Internal Medicine* 149 (2008): 100–108.

40 Kees van Grootheest, Linda de Fraaf, and Lolkje T. W. de Jong-van den Berg, "Consumer Adverse Drug Reaction Reporting: A New Step in Pharmacovigilance?" *Drug Safety* 26 (2003): 211–17.

41 See http://www.consumerreports.org/health/best-buy-drugs/index.htm.

42 Jerry Avorn, "Debate about Funding Comparative-Effectiveness Research," *New England Journal of Medicine* 360 (2009): 1927–29.

43 Ibid.

44 Silvio Garattini and Iain Chalmers, "Patients and the Public Deserve Big Changes in Evaluation of Drugs," *British Medical Journal* 338 (2009): b1025, http://www.bmj.com/cgi/content/extract/338/mar31_3/b1025?papetoc.

45 Avorn, "Debate about Funding."

46 Salomeh Keyhani, Marie Diener-West, and Neil Powe, "Do Drug Prices Reflect Development Time and Government Investment?" *Medical Care* 43 (2005): 753–62.

47 Garattini and Chalmers, "Patients and the Public."

48 Angell, *Truth About the Drug Companies*, 240.

49 *Consumer Reports*, "Best Buy Drugs—the Proton Pump Inhibitors," http://www.consumerreports.org/health/resources/pdf/best-buy-drugs/PPIsUPdate-2pager-Feb07.pdf.

50 Reed Abelson and Andrew Pollack, "Medicare Widens Drugs It Accepts for Cancer," *New York Times*, January 26, 2009, http://www.nytimes.com/2009/01/27/health/27cancer.html?_r=1.

51 Garattini and Chalmers, "Patients and the Public."

52 Donald W. Light, "Basic Research Funds to Discover Important New Drugs: Who Contributes How Much?" in *Monitoring Financial Flows for Health Research 2005: Behind the Global Numbers*, Mary Anne Burke and Andrés de Francisco, eds. (Geneva: Global Forum for Health Research, 2006), chap. 3; Donald W. Light, "Misleading Congress about Drug Development," *Journal of Health Politics, Policy and Law* 32 (2007): 895–913.

53 Merrill Goozner, *The $800 Million Pill: The Truth Behind the Cost of New Drugs* (Berkeley: University of California Press, 2004).

54 Kaiser Family Foundation, *Prescription Drug Trends*, Fact Sheet #3057-07, September 2008.

55 Congressional Budget Office, *Research and Development in the Pharmaceutical Industry*, 2006.

56 On this point, see especially Angell, *Truth About the Drug Companies*.

57 Donald W. Light and Joel Lexchin, "Foreign Free Riders and the High Price of US Medicines," *British Medical Journal* 331 (2005): 958–60.

58 Dean Baker and Noriko Chatani, *Promoting Good Ideas on Drugs: The Relative Efficiency of Patent and Public Support for Bio-Medical Research* (Washington, DC: Center for Economic Policy and Research, 2002), http://www.cepr.net/index.php/ publications/reports/promoting-good-ideas-on-drugs-are-patents-the-best-way/.

59 Angell, *Truth About the Drug Companies*, 249.

60 European Commission for Competition, *Pharmaceutical Sector Inquiry: Preliminary Report* (Brussels: European Commission for Competition, 2008).

Contributors

HOWARD BRODY, MD, PhD, is John P. McGovern Centennial Chair in Family Medicine and director, Institute for the Medical Humanities, at the University of Texas Medical Branch in Galveston. He is the author of *The Future of Bioethics* (Oxford University Press, 2009) and *Hooked: Ethics, the Medical Profession, and the Pharmaceutical Industry* (Rowman & Littlefield, 2007).

PETER CONRAD is the Harry Coplan Professor of Social Sciences at Brandeis University. His most recent book is *The Medicalization of Society: On the Transformation of Human Conditions into Treatable Disorders* (Johns Hopkins University Press, 2007). His current research focuses on ADHD, behavioral difference, and life success.

ALLAN V. HORWITZ is professor of sociology and dean of Social and Behavioral Science at Rutgers University. He is the author of over 100 articles and chapters on various aspects of the sociology of mental illness. His most recent books are *The Loss of Sadness* (Oxford University Press with Jerome Wakefield) and *Diagnosis, Therapy, and Evidence* (Rutgers University Press with Gerald Grob).

DONALD W. LIGHT is a professor at the University of Medicine & Dentistry of New Jersey, School of Osteopathic Medicine. A medical and economic sociologist, Light conducts policy research on the efficacy, safety, and affordability of medicines. His work has been published in *The Lancet*, the *British Medical Journal*, *PLoS-Medicine*, *Vaccine*, the *Journal of Health Economics*, the *Journal of Health Politics, Policy and Law*, the *American Journal of Bioethics*, and *Health Affairs*.

CHERYL STULTS received her PhD in Sociology from Brandeis University in 2009. Her research interests include women's health, illness on the Internet, and public perceptions of risk. She is currently continuing her research and writing on the process of risk scares in society.